Skill Checklists for

Fundamentals
of Nursing

THE ART AND SCIENCE OF NURSING CARE

Skill Checklists for

Fundamentals of Nursing

THE ART AND SCIENCE OF NURSING CARE

SEVENTH EDITION

Carol R. Taylor, PhD, MSN, RN
Center for Clinical Bioethics
Professor of Nursing
Georgetown University
Washington, DC

Carol Lillis, MSN, RN
Faculty Emerita, Assistant to the Provost
Delaware County Community College
Media, Pennsylvania

Priscilla LeMone, DSN, RN, FAAN
Associate Professor Emerita, Sinclair School of Nursing
University of Missouri-Columbia
Columbia, Missouri
Adjunct Associate Professor, College of Nursing
The Ohio State University
Columbus, Ohio

Pamela Lynn, MSN, RN
Instructor
School of Nursing
Gwynedd-Mercy College
Gwynedd Valley, Pennsylvania

Marilee LeBon, BA
Editor
Brigantine, New Jersey

Wolters Kluwer | Lippincott Williams & Wilkins
Health
Philadelphia · Baltimore · New York · London
Buenos Aires · Hong Kong · Sydney · Tokyo

Executive Acquisitions Editor: Carrie Brandon
Senior Product Manager: Betsy Gentzler
Design Coordinator: Holly McLaughlin
Manufacturing Coordinator: Karin Duffield
Prepress Vendor: Aptara, Inc.

7th edition

9 8 7 6 5 4 3 2 1

Printed in the United States of America.

ISBN: 978-0-7817-9385-8

Care has been taken to confirm the accuracy of the information presented and to describe generally accepted practices. However, the authors, editors, and publisher are not responsible for errors or omissions or for any consequences from application of the information in this book and make no warranty, expressed or implied, with respect to the currency, completeness, or accuracy of the contents of the publication. Application of this information in a particular situation remains the professional responsibility of the practitioner; the clinical treatments described and recommended may not be considered absolute and universal recommendations.

The authors, editors, and publisher have exerted every effort to ensure that drug selection and dosage set forth in this text are in accordance with the current recommendations and practice at the time of publication. However, in view of ongoing research, changes in government regulations, and the constant flow of information relating to drug therapy and drug reactions, the reader is urged to check the package insert for each drug for any change in indications and dosage and for added warnings and precautions. This is particularly important when the recommended agent is a new or infrequently employed drug.

Some drugs and medical devices presented in this publication have Food and Drug Administration (FDA) clearance for limited use in restricted research settings. It is the responsibility of the health care provider to ascertain the FDA status of each drug or device planned for use in his or her clinical practice.

LWW.com

Introduction

Developing clinical competency is an important challenge for each fundamentals nursing student. To facilitate the mastery of nursing skills, we are happy to provide skill checklists for each skill included in *Fundamentals of Nursing: The Art and Science of Nursing Care*, Seventh Edition. Students can use the checklists to facilitate self-evaluation, and faculty will find them useful in measuring and recording student performance. Three-hole-punched and perforated, these checklists can be easily reproduced and brought to the simulation laboratory or clinical area.

The checklists follow each step of the skill to provide a complete evaluative tool. They are designed to record an evaluation of each step of the procedure.

- Checkmark in the "Excellent" column denotes mastering the procedure.
- Checkmark in the "Satisfactory" column indicates use of the recommended technique.
- Checkmark in the "Needs Practice" column indicates use of some but not all of each recommended technique.

The Comments section allows you to highlight suggestions that will improve skills. Space is available at the top of each checklist to record a final pass/fail evaluation, date, and the signature of the student and evaluating faculty member.

List of Skills by Chapter

List of Skills in Alphabetical Order

Skill Checklists for Fundamentals of Nursing:
The Art and Science of Nursing Care, 7th edition

Name _____ Date _____

Unit _____ Position _____

Instructor/Evaluator: _____ Position _____

SKILL 24-1

Assessing Body Temperature

Excellent	Satisfactory	Needs Practice	**Goal:** The patient's temperature is assessed accurately without injury and the patient experiences only minimal discomfort.	**Comments**
___	___	___	1. Check medical order or nursing care plan for frequency of measurement and route. More frequent temperature measurement may be appropriate based on nursing judgment. Bring necessary equipment to the bedside stand or overbed table.	
___	___	___	2. Perform hand hygiene and put on PPE, if indicated.	
___	___	___	3. Identify the patient.	
___	___	___	4. Close curtains around bed and close door to room if possible. Discuss procedure with patient and assess patient's ability to assist with the procedure.	
___	___	___	5. Ensure the electronic or digital thermometer is in working condition.	
___	___	___	6. Put on gloves if appropriate or indicated.	
___	___	___	7. Select the appropriate site based on previous assessment data.	
___	___	___	8. Follow the steps as outlined below for the appropriate type of thermometer.	
___	___	___	9. When measurement is completed, remove gloves, if worn. Remove additional PPE, if used. Perform hand hygiene.	
			Measuring a Tympanic Membrane Temperature	
___	___	___	10. If necessary, push the "on" button and wait for the "ready" signal on the unit.	
___	___	___	11. Slide disposable cover onto the tympanic probe.	
___	___	___	12. *Insert the probe snugly into the external ear using gentle but firm pressure, angling the thermometer toward the patient's jaw line. Pull pinna up and back to straighten the ear canal in an adult.*	
___	___	___	13. Activate the unit by pushing the trigger button. The reading is immediate (usually within 2 seconds). Note the reading.	
___	___	___	14. Discard the probe cover in an appropriate receptacle by pushing the probe-release button or use rim of cover to remove from probe. Replace the thermometer in its charger, if necessary.	

Assessing Body Temperature (Continued)

Excellent	Satisfactory	Needs Practice		Comments
			Assessing Oral Temperature	
___	___	___	10. Remove the electronic unit from the charging unit, and remove the probe from within the recording unit.	
___	___	___	11. Cover thermometer probe with disposable probe cover and slide it on until it snaps into place.	
___	___	___	12. *Place the probe beneath the patient's tongue in the posterior sublingual pocket. Ask the patient to close his or her lips around the probe.*	
___	___	___	13. *Continue to hold the probe until you hear a beep. Note the temperature reading.*	
___	___	___	14. Remove the probe from the patient's mouth. Dispose of the probe cover by holding the probe over an appropriate receptacle and pressing the probe release button.	
___	___	___	15. Return the thermometer probe to the storage place within the unit. Return the electronic unit to the charging unit, if appropriate.	
			Assessing Rectal Temperature	
___	___	___	10. Adjust the bed to a comfortable working height, usually elbow height of the caregiver (VISN 8, 2009). Put on non-sterile gloves.	
___	___	___	11. Assist the patient to a side-lying position. Pull back the covers enough to expose only the buttocks.	
___	___	___	12. Remove the rectal probe from within the recording unit of the electronic thermometer. Cover the probe with a disposable probe cover and slide it into place until it snaps in place.	
___	___	___	13. *Lubricate about 1" of the probe with a water-soluble lubricant.*	
___	___	___	14. Reassure the patient. Separate the buttocks until the anal sphincter is clearly visible.	
___	___	___	15. *Insert the thermometer probe into the anus about 1.5" in an adult or 1" in a child.*	
___	___	___	16. Hold the probe in place until you hear a beep, then carefully remove the probe. Note the temperature reading on the display.	
___	___	___	17. Dispose of the probe cover by holding the probe over an appropriate waste receptacle and pressing the release button.	
___	___	___	18. Using toilet tissue, wipe the anus of any feces or excess lubricant. Dispose of the toilet tissue. Remove gloves and discard them.	

SKILL 24-1
Assessing Body Temperature (Continued)

Excellent	Satisfactory	Needs Practice		Comments
——	——	——	19. Cover the patient and help him or her to a position of comfort.	
——	——	——	20. Place the bed in the lowest position; elevate rails as needed.	
——	——	——	21. Return the thermometer to the charging unit.	
			Assessing Axillary Temperature	
——	——	——	10. Move the patient's clothing to expose only the axilla.	
——	——	——	11. Remove the probe from the recording unit of the electronic thermometer. Place a disposable probe cover on by sliding it on and snapping it securely.	
——	——	——	12. *Place the end of the probe in the center of the axilla. Have the patient bring the arm down and close to the body.*	
——	——	——	13. Hold the probe in place until you hear a beep, and then carefully remove the probe. Note the temperature reading.	
——	——	——	14. Cover the patient and help him or her to a position of comfort.	
——	——	——	15. Dispose of the probe cover by holding the probe over an appropriate waste receptacle and pushing the release button.	
——	——	——	16. Place the bed in the lowest position and elevate rails as needed. Leave the patient clean and comfortable.	
——	——	——	17. Return the electronic thermometer to the charging unit.	
			Assessing Temporal Artery Temperature	
——	——	——	10. Brush the patient's hair aside if it is covering the temporal artery area.	
——	——	——	11. Apply a probe cover.	
——	——	——	12. Hold the thermometer like a remote, with your thumb on the red "ON" button. Place the probe flush on the center of the forehead, with the body of the instrument sideways (not straight up and down), so it is not in the patient's face.	
——	——	——	13. Depress the "ON" button. Keep the button depressed throughout the measurement.	
——	——	——	14. Slowly slide the probe straight across the forehead, midline, to the hairline. The thermometer will click; fast clicking indicates a rise to a higher temperature, slow clicking indicates the instrument is still scanning, but not finding any higher temperature.	

SKILL 24-1

Assessing Body Temperature *(Continued)*

Excellent	Satisfactory	Needs Practice		Comments
——	——	——	15. Brush hair aside if it is covering the ear, exposing the area of the neck under the ear lobe. Lift the probe from the forehead and touch on the neck just behind the ear lobe, in the depression just below the mastoid.	
——	——	——	16. Release the button and read the thermometer measurement.	
——	——	——	17. Hold the thermometer over a waste receptacle. Gently push the probe cover with your thumb against the proximal edge to dispose of probe cover.	
——	——	——	18. Instrument will automatically turn off in 30 seconds, or press and release the power button.	

Skill Checklists for Fundamentals of Nursing:
The Art and Science of Nursing Care, 7th edition

Name _____   Date _____

Unit _____   Position _____

Instructor/Evaluator: _____   Position _____

SKILL 24-2
Assessing a Peripheral Pulse by Palpation

Goal: The patient's pulse is assessed accurately without injury and the patient experiences only minimal discomfort.

Excellent	Satisfactory	Needs Practice		Comments
——	——	——	1. Check medical order or nursing care plan for frequency of pulse assessment. More frequent pulse measurement may be appropriate based on nursing judgment.	
——	——	——	2. Perform hand hygiene and put on PPE, if indicated.	
——	——	——	3. Identify the patient.	
——	——	——	4. Close curtains around bed and close door to room if possible. Discuss procedure with patient and assess patient's ability to assist with the procedure.	
——	——	——	5. Put on gloves as appropriate.	
——	——	——	6. Select the appropriate peripheral site based on assessment data.	
——	——	——	7. Move the patient's clothing to expose only the site chosen.	
——	——	——	8. Place your first, second, and third fingers over the artery. *Lightly compress the artery so pulsations can be felt and counted.*	
——	——	——	9. Using a watch with a second hand, count the number of pulsations felt for 30 seconds. Multiply this number by 2 to calculate the rate for 1 minute. *If the rate, rhythm, or amplitude of the pulse is abnormal in any way, palpate and count the pulse for 1 minute.*	
——	——	——	10. Note the rhythm and amplitude of the pulse.	
——	——	——	11. When measurement is completed, remove gloves, if worn. Cover the patient and help him or her to a position of comfort.	
——	——	——	12. Remove additional PPE, if used. Perform hand hygiene.	

Skill Checklists for Fundamentals of Nursing:
The Art and Science of Nursing Care, 7th edition

Name _____   Date _____

Unit _____   Position _____

Instructor/Evaluator: _____   Position _____

SKILL 24-3

Assessing Respiration

Goal: The patient's respirations are assessed accurately without injury and the patient experiences only minimal discomfort.

Excellent	Satisfactory	Needs Practice		Comments
___	___	___	1. *While your fingers are still in place for the pulse measurement, after counting the pulse rate, observe the patient's respirations.*	
___	___	___	2. Note the rise and fall of the patient's chest.	
___	___	___	3. Using a watch with a second hand, count the number of respirations for 30 seconds. Multiply this number by 2 to calculate the respiratory rate per minute.	
___	___	___	4. *If respirations are abnormal in any way, count the respirations for at least 1 full minute.*	
___	___	___	5. Note the depth and rhythm of the respirations.	
___	___	___	6. When measurement is completed, remove gloves, if worn. Cover the patient and help him or her to a position of comfort.	
___	___	___	7. Remove additional PPE, if used. Perform hand hygiene.	

Skill Checklists for Fundamentals of Nursing:
The Art and Science of Nursing Care, 7th edition

Name _____ Date _____

Unit _____ Position _____

Instructor/Evaluator: _____ Position _____

			SKILL 24-4	

Assessing a Brachial Artery Blood Pressure

Excellent	Satisfactory	Needs Practice	**Goal:** The patient's blood pressure is measured accurately with minimal discomfort to the patient.	**Comments**
— — —			1. Check physician's order or nursing care plan for frequency of blood pressure measurement. More frequent measurement may be appropriate based on nursing judgment.	
— — —			2. Perform hand hygiene and put on PPE, if indicated.	
— — —			3. Identify the patient.	
— — —			4. Close curtains around bed and close door to room if possible. Discuss procedure with patient and assess patient's ability to assist with the procedure. Validate that the patient has relaxed for several minutes.	
— — —			5. Put on gloves, if appropriate or indicated.	
— — —			6. Select the appropriate arm for application of the cuff.	
— — —			7. Have the patient assume a comfortable lying or sitting position with the forearm supported at the level of the heart and the palm of the hand upward. If the measurement is taken in the supine position, support the arm with a pillow. In the sitting position, support the arm yourself or by using the bedside table. If the patient is sitting, have the patient sit back in the chair so that the chair supports his or her back. In addition, make sure the patient keeps the legs uncrossed.	
— — —			8. Expose the brachial artery by removing garments, or move a sleeve, if it is not too tight, above the area where the cuff will be placed.	
— — —			9. Palpate the location of the brachial artery. *Center the bladder of the cuff over the brachial artery, about midway on the arm, so that the lower edge of the cuff is about 2.5 to 5 cm (1″–2″) above the inner aspect of the elbow. Line the artery marking on the cuff up with the patient's brachial artery.* The tubing should extend from the edge of the cuff nearer the patient's elbow.	
— — —			10. Wrap the cuff around the arm smoothly and snugly, and fasten it. Do not allow any clothing to interfere with the proper placement of the cuff.	
— — —			11. Check that the needle on the aneroid gauge is within the zero mark. If using a mercury manometer, check to see that the manometer is in the vertical position and that the mercury is within the zero level with the gauge at eye level.	

SKILL 24-4
Assessing a Brachial Artery Blood Pressure *(Continued)*

Excellent	Satisfactory	Needs Practice		Comments

Estimating Systolic Pressure

_____ _____ _____ 12. Palpate the pulse at the brachial or radial artery by pressing gently with the fingertips.

_____ _____ _____ 13. Tighten the screw valve on the air pump.

_____ _____ _____ 14. *Inflate the cuff while continuing to palpate the artery. Note the point on the gauge where the pulse disappears.*

_____ _____ _____ 15. Deflate the cuff and wait 1 minute.

Obtaining Blood Pressure Measurement

_____ _____ _____ 16. Assume a position that is no more than 3 feet away from the gauge.

_____ _____ _____ 17. Place the stethoscope earpieces in your ears. Direct the earpieces forward into the canal and not against the ear itself.

_____ _____ _____ 18. Place the bell or diaphragm of the stethoscope firmly but with as little pressure as possible over the brachial artery. Do not allow the stethoscope to touch clothing or the cuff.

_____ _____ _____ 19. Pump the pressure 30-mm Hg above the point at which the systolic pressure was palpated and estimated. Open the valve on the manometer and allow air to escape slowly (allowing the gauge to drop 2-3 mm per second).

_____ _____ _____ 20. *Note the point on the gauge at which the first faint, but clear, sound appears that slowly increases in intensity. Note this number as the systolic pressure. Read the pressure to the closest 2 mm Hg.*

_____ _____ _____ 21. Do not reinflate the cuff once the air is being released to recheck the systolic pressure reading.

_____ _____ _____ 22. *Note the point at which the sound completely disappears.*

_____ _____ _____ 23. Allow the remaining air to escape quickly. Repeat any suspicious reading, but wait at least 1 minute. Deflate the cuff completely between attempts to check the blood pressure.

_____ _____ _____ 24. When measurement is completed, remove the cuff. Remove gloves, if worn. Cover the patient and help him or her to a position of comfort.

_____ _____ _____ 25. Remove additional PPE, if used. Perform hand hygiene.

_____ _____ _____ 26. Clean the diaphragm of the stethoscope with the alcohol wipe. Clean and store the sphygmomanometer, according to facility policy.

Skill Checklists for Fundamentals of Nursing:
The Art and Science of Nursing Care, 7th edition

Name _____   Date _____

Unit _____   Position _____

Instructor/Evaluator: _____   Position _____

Excellent	Satisfactory	Needs Practice	SKILL 26-1 **Applying an Extremity Restraint**	
			Goal: The patient is constrained by the restraint, remains free from injury, and the restraint does not interfere with therapeutic devices.	**Comments**
――	――	――	1. Determine need for restraints. Assess patient's physical condition, behavior, and mental status.	
――	――	――	2. Confirm agency policy for application of restraints. *Secure an order from the primary care provider, or validate that the order has been obtained within the past 24 hours.*	
――	――	――	3. Perform hand hygiene and put on PPE, if indicated.	
――	――	――	4. Identify the patient.	
――	――	――	5. Explain reason for use to patient and family. Clarify how care will be given and how needs will be met. Explain that restraint is a temporary measure.	
――	――	――	6. Include the patient's family and/or significant others in the plan of care.	
――	――	――	7. Apply restraint according to manufacturer's directions:	
――	――	――	a. Choose the least restrictive type of device that allows the greatest possible degree of mobility.	
――	――	――	b. Pad bony prominences.	
――	――	――	c. Wrap the restraint around the extremity with the soft part in contact with the skin. If hand mitt is being used, pull over hand with cushion to the palmar aspect of hand. Secure in place with the Velcro® straps.	
――	――	――	8. *Ensure that two fingers can be inserted between the restraint and patient's wrist or ankle.*	
――	――	――	9. Maintain restrained extremity in normal anatomic position. *Use a quick-release knot to tie the restraint to the bed frame, not side rail. The restraint may also be attached to chair frame.* The site should not be readily accessible to patient.	
――	――	――	10. Remove PPE, if used. Perform hand hygiene.	
――	――	――	11. Assess the patient at least every hour or according to facility policy. Assessment should include: the placement of the restraint, neurovascular assessment of the affected extremity, and skin integrity. In addition, assess for signs of sensory deprivation such as increased sleeping, daydreaming, anxiety, panic, and hallucinations.	

Excellent	Satisfactory	Needs Practice	SKILL 26-1 **Applying an Extremity Restraint** *(Continued)*	Comments
——	——	——	12. *Remove restraint at least every 2 hours, or according to agency policy and patient need.* Perform range-of-motion exercises.	
——	——	——	13. Evaluate patient for continued need of restraint. Reapply restraint only if continued need is evident and order is still valid.	
——	——	——	14. Reassure patient at regular intervals. Provide continued explanation of rationale for interventions, reorientation if necessary, and plan of care. *Keep call bell within easy reach.*	

Skill Checklists for Fundamentals of Nursing:
The Art and Science of Nursing Care, 7th edition

Name _____   Date _____

Unit _____   Position _____

Instructor/Evaluator: _____   Position _____

SKILL 27-1

Performing Hand Hygiene Using Soap and Water (Handwashing)

Goal: The hands will be free of visible soiling and transient microorganisms will be eliminated.

Excellent	Satisfactory	Needs Practice		Comments
——	——	——	1. Gather the necessary supplies. Stand in front of the sink. Do not allow your clothing to touch the sink during the washing procedure.	
——	——	——	2. Remove jewelry, if possible, and secure in a safe place. A plain wedding band may remain in place.	
——	——	——	3. Turn on water and adjust force. Regulate the temperature until the water is warm.	
——	——	——	4. Wet the hands and wrist area. Keep hands lower than elbows to allow water to flow toward fingertips.	
——	——	——	5. Use about 1 teaspoon of liquid soap from dispenser or rinse bar of soap and lather thoroughly. Cover all areas of hands with the soap product. Rinse soap bar again and return to soap rack.	
——	——	——	6. With firm rubbing and circular motions, wash the palms and backs of the hands, each finger, the areas between the fingers, and the knuckles, wrists, and forearms. *Wash at least 1 inch above area of contamination.* If hands are not visibly soiled, wash to 1 inch above the wrists	
——	——	——	7. Continue this friction motion for at least 15 seconds.	
——	——	——	8. Use fingernails of the opposite hand or a clean orangewood stick to clean under fingernails.	
——	——	——	9. Rinse thoroughly with water flowing toward fingertips.	
——	——	——	10. Pat hands dry with a paper towel, beginning with the fingers and moving upward toward forearms, and discard it immediately. Use another clean towel to turn off the faucet. Discard towel immediately without touching other clean hand.	
——	——	——	11. Use oil-free lotion on hands, if desired.	

Skill Checklists for Fundamentals of Nursing:
The Art and Science of Nursing Care, 7th edition

Name _____   Date _____

Unit _____   Position _____

Instructor/Evaluator: _____   Position _____

Excellent	Satisfactory	Needs Practice	SKILL 27-2 **Using Personal Protective Equipment**	
			Goal: The transmission of microorganisms is prevented.	**Comments**
____	____	____	1. Check medical record and nursing plan of care for type of precautions and review precautions in infection-control manual.	
____	____	____	2. Plan nursing activities before entering patient's room.	
____	____	____	3. Perform hand hygiene.	
____	____	____	4. Provide instruction about precautions to patient, family members, and visitors.	
____	____	____	5. Put on gown, gloves, mask, and protective eyewear, based on the type of exposure anticipated and category of isolation precautions.	
____	____	____	a. Put on the gown, with the opening in the back. Tie gown securely at neck and waist.	
____	____	____	b. Put on the mask or respirator over your nose, mouth, and chin. Secure ties or elastic bands at the middle of the head and neck. If respirator is used, perform a fit check. Inhale; the respirator should collapse. Exhale; air should not leak out.	
____	____	____	c. Put on goggles. Place over eyes and adjust to fit. Alternately, a face shield could be used to take the place of the mask and goggles.	
____	____	____	d. Put on clean disposable gloves. Extend gloves to cover the cuffs of the gown.	
____	____	____	6. Identify the patient. Explain the procedure to the patient. Continue with patient care as appropriate.	
			Remove PPE	
____	____	____	7. Remove PPE: Except for respirator, remove PPE at the doorway or in anteroom. Remove respirator after leaving the patient room and closing door.	
____	____	____	a. If impervious gown has been tied in front of the body at the waistline, untie waist strings before removing gloves.	
____	____	____	b. Grasp the outside of one glove with the opposite gloved hand and peel off, turning the glove inside out as you pull it off. Hold the removed glove in the remaining gloved hand.	

SKILL 27-2

Using Personal Protective Equipment *(Continued)*

Excellent	Satisfactory	Needs Practice		Comments
——	——	——	c. Slide fingers of ungloved hand under the remaining glove at the wrist, taking care not to touch the outer surface of the glove.	
——	——	——	d. Peel off the glove over the first glove, containing the one glove inside the other. Discard in appropriate container.	
——	——	——	e. To remove the goggles or face shield: Handle by the headband or ear pieces. Lift away from the face. Place in designated receptacle for reprocessing or in an appropriate waste container.	
——	——	——	f. To remove gown: Unfasten ties, if at the neck and back. Allow the gown to fall away from shoulders. Touching only the inside of the gown, pull away from the torso. Keeping hands on the inner surface of the gown, pull from arms. Turn gown inside out. Fold or roll into a bundle and discard.	
——	——	——	g. To remove mask or respirator: Grasp the neck ties or elastic, then top ties or elastic and remove. Take care to avoid touching front of mask or respirator. Discard in waste container. If using a respirator, save for future use in the designated area.	
——	——	——	8. Perform hand hygiene immediately after removing all PPE.	

Skill Checklists for Fundamentals of Nursing:
The Art and Science of Nursing Care, 7th edition

Name _____ Date _____

Unit _____ Position _____

Instructor/Evaluator: _____ Position _____

SKILL 27-3

Preparing a Sterile Field and Adding Sterile Items to a Sterile Field

Goal: The sterile field is created without contamination and the patient remains free of exposure to potential infection-causing microorganisms.

Excellent	Satisfactory	Needs Practice		Comments
____	____	____	1. Perform hand hygiene and put on PPE, if indicated.	
____	____	____	2. Identify the patient. Explain the procedure to the patient.	
			Preparing a Sterile Field	
____	____	____	3. Check that packaged sterile drape is dry and unopened. Also, note expiration date, making sure that the date is still valid.	
____	____	____	4. Select a work area that is waist level or higher.	
____	____	____	5. Open sterile wrapped drape or commercially prepared kit.	
			For a Prepackaged Sterile Drape	
____	____	____	a. Open the outer covering of the drape. Remove sterile drape, lifting it carefully by its corners. Hold away from body and above the waist and work surface.	
____	____	____	b. Continue to hold only by the corners. Allow the drape to unfold, away from your body and any other surface.	
____	____	____	c. Position the drape on the work surface with the moisture-proof side down. This would be the shiny or blue side. Avoid touching any other surface or object with the drape. If any portion of the drape hangs off the work surface, that part of the drape is considered contaminated.	
			For a Commercially Prepared Kit or Tray	
____	____	____	a. Open the outside cover of the package and remove the kit or tray. Place in the center of the work surface, with the topmost flap positioned on the far side of the package.	
____	____	____	b. Reach around the package and grasp the outer surface of the end of the topmost flap, holding no more than 1 inch from the border of the flap. Pull open away from the body, keeping the arm outstretched and away from the inside of the wrapper. Allow the wrapper to lie flat on the work surface.	

SKILL 27-3

Preparing a Sterile Field and Adding Sterile Items to a Sterile Field *(Continued)*

Excellent	Satisfactory	Needs Practice		Comments

c. Reach around the package and grasp the outer surface of the first side flap, holding no more than 1 inch from the border of the flap. Pull open to the side of the package, keeping the arm outstretched and away from the inside of the wrapper. Allow the wrapper to lie flat on the work surface.

d. Reach around the package and grasp the outer surface of the remaining side flap, holding no more than 1 inch from the border of the flap. Pull open to the side of the package, keeping the arm outstretched and away from the inside of the wrapper. Allow the wrapper to lie flat on the work surface.

e. Stand away from the package and work surface. Grasp the outer surface of the remaining flap closest to the body, holding not more than 1 inch from the border of the flap. Pull the flap back toward the body, keeping arm outstretched and away from the inside of the wrapper. Keep this hand in place. Use other hand to grasp the wrapper on the underside (the side that is down to the work surface). Position the wrapper so that when flat, edges are on the work surface, and do not hang down over sides of work surface. Allow the wrapper to lie flat on the work surface.

f. The outer wrapper of the package has become a sterile field with the packaged supplies in the center. Do not touch or reach over the sterile field.

Adding Items to a Sterile Field

6. Place additional sterile items on field as needed.

To Add an Agency-Wrapped and Sterilized Item

a. Hold agency-wrapped item in the dominant hand, with top flap opening away from the body. With other hand, reach around the package and unfold top flap and both sides.

b. Keep a secure hold on item through the wrapper with the dominant hand. Grasp the remaining flap of the wrapper closest to the body, taking care not to touch the inner surface of the wrapper or the item. Pull the flap back toward the wrist, so the wrapper covers the hand and wrist.

Excellent	Satisfactory	Needs Practice	SKILL 27-3 **Preparing a Sterile Field and Adding Sterile Items to a Sterile Field** *(Continued)*	Comments
——	——	——	c. Grasp all the corners of the wrapper together with the nondominant hand and pull back toward wrist, covering hand and wrist. Hold in place.	
——	——	——	d. Hold the item 6 inches above the surface of the sterile field and drop onto the field. Be careful to avoid touching the surface or other items or dropping onto the 1-inch border.	
			To Add a Commercially Wrapped and Sterilized Item	
——	——	——	a. Hold package in one hand. Pull back top cover with other hand. Alternately, carefully peel the edges apart using both hands.	
——	——	——	b. After top cover or edges are partially separated, hold the item 6 inches above the surface of the sterile field. Continue opening the package and drop the item onto the field. Be careful to avoid touching the surface or other items or dropping onto the 1-inch border.	
——	——	——	c. Discard wrapper.	
			To Add a Sterile Solution	
——	——	——	a. Obtain appropriate solution and check expiration date.	
——	——	——	b. Open solution container according to directions and *place cap on table away from the field with edges up.*	
——	——	——	c. Hold bottle outside the edge of the sterile field with the label side facing the palm of your hand and prepare to pour from a height of 4 to 6 inches (10 to 15 cm). The tip of the bottle should never touch a sterile container or field.	
——	——	——	d. Pour required amount of solution steadily into sterile container previously added to sterile field and positioned at side of sterile field or onto dressings. *Avoid splashing any liquid.*	
——	——	——	e. Touch only the outside of the lid when recapping. Label solution with date and time of opening.	
——	——	——	7. Continue with the procedure as indicated.	
——	——	——	8. When procedure is completed, remove PPE, if used. Perform hand hygiene.	

Skill Checklists for Fundamentals of Nursing:
The Art and Science of Nursing Care, 7th edition

Name _____   Date _____

Unit _____   Position _____

Instructor/Evaluator: _____   Position _____

Excellent	Satisfactory	Needs Practice	SKILL 27-4 **Putting on Sterile Gloves and Removing Soiled Gloves**	Comments
			Goal: The gloves are applied and removed without contamination.	
——	——	——	1. Perform hand hygiene and put on PPE, if indicated.	
——	——	——	2. Identify the patient. Explain the procedure to the patient.	
			Putting on Sterile Gloves	
——	——	——	3. Check that the sterile glove package is dry and unopened. Also, note expiration date, making sure that the date is still valid.	
——	——	——	4. Place sterile glove package on clean, dry surface at or above your waist.	
——	——	——	5. Open the outside wrapper by carefully peeling the top layer back. Remove inner package, handling only the outside of it.	
——	——	——	6. Place the inner package on the work surface with the side labeled "cuff end" closest to the body.	
——	——	——	7. Carefully open the inner package. Fold open the top flap, then the bottom and sides. Take care not to touch the inner surface of the package or the gloves.	
——	——	——	8. With the thumb and forefinger of the nondominant hand, grasp the folded cuff of the glove for dominant hand, touching only the exposed inside of the glove.	
——	——	——	9. Keeping the hands above the waistline, lift and hold the glove up and off the inner package with fingers down. *Be careful it does not touch any unsterile object.*	
——	——	——	10. Carefully insert dominant hand palm up into glove and pull glove on. Leave the cuff folded until the opposite hand is gloved.	
——	——	——	11. Hold the thumb of the gloved hand outward. Place the fingers of the gloved hand inside the cuff of the remaining glove. Lift it from the wrapper, taking care not to touch anything with the gloves or hands.	

Excellent	Satisfactory	Needs Practice	SKILL 27-4 **Putting on Sterile Gloves and Removing Soiled Gloves** *(Continued)*	
				Comments
——	——	——	12. Carefully insert nondominant hand into glove. Pull the glove on, taking care that the skin does not touch any of the outer surfaces of the gloves.	
——	——	——	13. *Slide the fingers of one hand under the cuff of the other and fully extend the cuff down the arm, touching only the sterile outside of the glove. Repeat for the remaining hand.*	
——	——	——	14. *Adjust gloves on both hands if necessary, touching only sterile areas with other sterile areas.*	
——	——	——	15. Continue with procedure as indicated.	
			Removing Soiled Gloves	
——	——	——	16. Use dominant hand to grasp the opposite glove near cuff end on the outside exposed area. Remove it by pulling it off, inverting it as it is pulled, keeping the contaminated area on the inside. Hold the removed glove in the remaining gloved hand.	
——	——	——	17. Slide fingers of ungloved hand between the remaining glove and the wrist. **Take care to avoid touching the outside surface of the glove.** Remove it by pulling it off, inverting it as it is pulled, keeping the contaminated area on the inside, and securing the first glove inside the second.	
——	——	——	18. Discard gloves in appropriate container. Remove additional PPE, if used. Perform hand hygiene.	

Skill Checklists for Fundamentals of Nursing:
The Art and Science of Nursing Care, 7th edition

Name _____ Date _____

Unit _____ Position _____

Instructor/Evaluator: _____ Position _____

SKILL 29-1

Administering Oral Medications

Goal: The patient will swallow the prescribed medication at the proper time.

Comments

Excellent	Satisfactory	Needs Practice		
——	——	——	1. Gather equipment. Check each medication order against the original in the medical record, according to facility policy. Clarify any inconsistencies. Check the patient's chart for allergies.	
——	——	——	2. Know the actions, special nursing considerations, safe dose ranges, purpose of administration, and adverse effects of the medications to be administered. Consider the appropriateness of the medication for this patient.	
——	——	——	3. Perform hand hygiene.	
——	——	——	4. Move the medication cart to the outside of the patient's room or prepare for administration in the medication area.	
——	——	——	5. Unlock the medication cart or drawer. Enter pass code into computer and scan employee identification, if required.	
——	——	——	6. *Prepare medications for one patient at a time.*	
——	——	——	7. Read the CMAR/MAR and select the proper medication from the patient's medication drawer or unit stock.	
——	——	——	8. Compare the label with the CMAR/MAR. Check expiration dates and perform calculations, if necessary. Scan the bar code on the package, if required.	
——	——	——	9. Prepare the required medications:	
——	——	——	a. *Unit dose packages:* Place unit dose-packaged medications in a disposable cup. **Do not open the wrapper until at the bedside.** Keep narcotics and medications that require special nursing assessments in a separate container.	
——	——	——	b. *Multidose containers:* When removing tablets or capsules from a multidose bottle, pour the necessary number into the bottle cap and then place the tablets or capsules in a medication cup. Break only scored tablets, if necessary, to obtain the proper dosage. Do not touch tablets or capsules with hands.	
——	——	——	c. *Liquid medication in multidose bottle:* When pouring liquid medications out of a multidose bottle, hold the bottle so the label is against the palm. Use the appropriate measuring device when pouring liquids, and read the amount of medication at the bottom of the meniscus at eye level. Wipe the lip of the bottle with a paper towel.	

SKILL 29-1

Administering Oral Medications *(Continued)*

Excellent	Satisfactory	Needs Practice		Comments
——	——	——	10. *When all medications for one patient have been prepared, recheck the labels with the CMAR/MAR before taking them to the patient. Replace any multidose containers in the patient's drawer or unit stock. Lock the medication cart before leaving it.*	
——	——	——	11. Transport medications to the patient's bedside carefully, and keep the medications in sight at all times.	
——	——	——	12. *Ensure that the patient receives the medications at the correct time.*	
——	——	——	13. Perform hand hygiene and put on PPE, if indicated.	
——	——	——	14. Identify the patient. Usually, the patient should be identified using two methods. Compare the information with the CMAR or MAR.	
——	——	——	a. Check the name and identification number on the patient's identification band.	
——	——	——	b. Ask the patient to state his or her name and birth date, based on facility policy.	
——	——	——	c. If the patient cannot identify him- or herself, verify the patient's identification with a staff member who knows the patient for the second source.	
——	——	——	15. *Scan the patient's bar code on the identification band, if required.*	
——	——	——	16. *Complete necessary assessments before administering medications. Check the patient's allergy bracelet or ask the patient about allergies. Explain the purpose and action of each medication to the patient.*	
——	——	——	17. Assist the patient to an upright or lateral position.	
——	——	——	18. Administer medications:	
——	——	——	a. Offer water or other permitted fluids with pills, capsules, tablets, and some liquid medications.	
——	——	——	b. Ask whether the patient prefers to take the medications by hand or in a cup.	
——	——	——	19. *Remain with the patient until each medication is swallowed. Never leave medication at the patient's bedside.*	
——	——	——	20. Assist the patient to a comfortable position. Remove PPE, if used. Perform hand hygiene.	
——	——	——	21. Document the administration of the medication immediately after administration.	
——	——	——	22. Evaluate patient's response to medication within appropriate time frame.	

Skill Checklists for Fundamentals of Nursing:
The Art and Science of Nursing Care, 7th edition

Name _____ Date _____

Unit _____ Position _____

Instructor/Evaluator: _____ Position _____

SKILL 29-2

Removing Medication from an Ampule

Goal: The proper dose of medication will be removed in a sterile manner, and will be free from glass shards.

Excellent	Satisfactory	Needs Practice		Comments
——	——	——	1. Gather equipment. Check the medication order against the original order in the medical record, according to facility policy. Clarify any inconsistencies. Check the patient's chart for allergies.	
——	——	——	2. Know the actions, special nursing considerations, safe dose ranges, purpose of administration, and adverse effects of the medications to be administered. Consider the appropriateness of the medication for this patient.	
——	——	——	3. Perform hand hygiene.	
——	——	——	4. Move the medication cart to the outside of the patient's room or prepare for administration in the medication area.	
——	——	——	5. Unlock the medication cart or drawer. Enter pass code and scan employee identification, if required.	
——	——	——	6. *Prepare medications for one patient at a time.*	
——	——	——	7. Read the CMAR/MAR and select the proper medication from the patient's medication drawer or unit stock.	
——	——	——	8. Compare the label with the CMAR/MAR. Check expiration dates and perform calculations, if necessary. Scan the bar code on the package, if required.	
——	——	——	9. Tap the stem of the ampule or twist your wrist quickly while holding the ampule vertically.	
——	——	——	10. Wrap a small gauze pad around the neck of the ampule.	
——	——	——	11. Use a snapping motion to break off the top of the ampule along the scored line at its neck. *Always break away from your body.*	
——	——	——	12. Attach filter needle to syringe. Remove the cap from the filter needle by pulling it straight off.	
——	——	——	13. Withdraw medication in the amount ordered plus a small amount more (approximately 30% more). *Do not inject air into the solution.* Use either of the following methods. *While inserting the filter needle into the ampule, be careful not to touch the rim.*	
——	——	——	a. Insert the tip of the needle into the ampule, which is upright on a flat surface, and withdraw fluid into the syringe. *Touch the plunger at the knob only.*	

SKILL 29-2

Removing Medication from an Ampule *(Continued)*

Excellent	Satisfactory	Needs Practice		Comments
——	——	——	b. Insert the tip of the needle into the ampule and invert the ampule. Keep the needle centered and not touching the sides of the ampule. Withdraw fluid into syringe. *Touch the plunger at the knob only.*	
——	——	——	14. Wait until the needle has been withdrawn to tap the syringe and expel the air carefully by pushing on the plunger. *Check the amount of medication in the syringe with the medication dose and discard any surplus according to facility policy.*	
——	——	——	15. *Recheck the label with the CMAR/MAR.*	
——	——	——	16. *Engage safety guard on filter needle and remove the needle. Discard the filter needle in a suitable container. Attach appropriate administration device to syringe.*	
——	——	——	17. Discard the ampule in a suitable container.	
——	——	——	18. Lock the medication cart before leaving it.	
——	——	——	19. Perform hand hygiene.	
——	——	——	20. Proceed with administration, based on prescribed route.	

Skill Checklists for Fundamentals of Nursing:
The Art and Science of Nursing Care, 7th edition

Name _____   Date _____

Unit _____   Position _____

Instructor/Evaluator: _____   Position _____

SKILL 29-3
Removing Medication From a Vial

Excellent	Satisfactory	Needs Practice	**Goal:** The proper dosage of medication is withdrawn into a syringe using sterile technique.	Comments
——	——	——	1. Gather equipment. Check the medication order against the original order in the medical record, according to facility policy.	
——	——	——	2. Know the actions, special nursing considerations, safe dose ranges, purpose of administration, and adverse effects of the medications to be administered. Consider the appropriateness of the medication for this patient.	
——	——	——	3. Perform hand hygiene.	
——	——	——	4. Move the medication cart to the outside of the patient's room or prepare for administration in the medication area.	
——	——	——	5. Unlock the medication cart or drawer. Enter pass code and scan employee identification, if required.	
——	——	——	6. *Prepare medications for one patient at a time.*	
——	——	——	7. Read the CMAR/MAR and select the proper medication from the patient's medication drawer or unit stock.	
——	——	——	8. Compare the label with the CMAR/MAR. Check expiration dates and perform calculations, if necessary. Scan the bar code on the package, if required.	
——	——	——	9. Remove the metal or plastic cap on the vial that protects the rubber stopper.	
——	——	——	10. *Swab the rubber top with the antimicrobial swab and allow to dry.*	
——	——	——	11. Remove the cap from the needle or blunt cannula by pulling it straight off. Touch the plunger at the knob only. Draw back an amount of air into the syringe that is equal to the specific dose of medication to be withdrawn. Some facilities require use of a filter needle when withdrawing premixed medication from multidose vials.	
——	——	——	12. Hold the vial on a flat surface. Pierce the rubber stopper in the center with the needle tip and inject the measured air into the space above the solution. Do not inject air into the solution.	
——	——	——	13. *Invert the vial. Keep the tip of the needle or blunt cannula below the fluid level.*	

Excellent	Satisfactory	Needs Practice		Comments
			SKILL 29-3 **Removing Medication From a Vial** *(Continued)*	
——	——	——	14. Hold the vial in one hand and use the other to withdraw the medication. Touch the plunger at the knob only. *Draw up the prescribed amount of medication while holding the syringe vertically and at eye level.*	
——	——	——	15. If any air bubbles accumulate in the syringe, tap the barrel of the syringe sharply and move the needle past the fluid into the air space to re-inject the air bubble into the vial. Return the needle tip to the solution and continue withdrawal of the medication.	
——	——	——	16. After the correct dose is withdrawn, remove the needle from the vial and carefully replace the cap over the needle. *If a filter needle has been used to draw up the medication, remove it and attach the appropriate administration device.* Some facilities require changing the needle, if one was used to withdraw the medication, before administering the medication.	
——	——	——	17. *Check the amount of medication in the syringe with the medication dose and discard any surplus.*	
——	——	——	18. *Recheck the label with the CMAR/MAR.*	
——	——	——	19. *If a multidose vial is being used, label the vial with the date and time opened, and store the vial containing the remaining medication according to facility policy.*	
——	——	——	20. Lock the medication cart before leaving it.	
——	——	——	21. Perform hand hygiene.	
——	——	——	22. Proceed with administration, based on prescribed route.	

Skill Checklists for Fundamentals of Nursing:
The Art and Science of Nursing Care, 7th edition

Name _____   Date _____

Unit _____   Position _____

Instructor/Evaluator: _____   Position _____

SKILL 29-4

Mixing Medications From Two Vials in One Syringe

Excellent	Satisfactory	Needs Practice	**Goal:** The proper dosage of medication is withdrawn into a syringe using sterile technique.	Comments
⎯	⎯	⎯	1. Gather equipment. Check medication order against the original order in the medical record, according to facility policy.	
⎯	⎯	⎯	2. Know the actions, special nursing considerations, safe dose ranges, purpose of administration, and adverse effects of the medications to be administered. Consider the appropriateness of the medication for this patient.	
⎯	⎯	⎯	3. Perform hand hygiene.	
⎯	⎯	⎯	4. Move the medication cart to the outside of the patient's room or prepare for administration in the medication area.	
⎯	⎯	⎯	5. Unlock the medication cart or drawer. Enter pass code and scan employee identification, if required.	
⎯	⎯	⎯	6. *Prepare medications for one patient at a time.*	
⎯	⎯	⎯	7. Read the CMAR/MAR and select the proper medications from the patient's medication drawer or unit stock.	
⎯	⎯	⎯	8. Compare the labels with the CMAR/MAR. Check expiration dates and perform calculations, if necessary. Scan the bar code on the package, if required.	
⎯	⎯	⎯	9. If necessary, remove the cap that protects the rubber stopper on each vial.	
⎯	⎯	⎯	10. *If medication is a suspension (e.g., NPH insulin), roll and agitate the vial to mix it well.*	
⎯	⎯	⎯	11. Cleanse the rubber tops with antimicrobial swabs.	
⎯	⎯	⎯	12. Remove cap from needle by pulling it straight off. Touch the plunger at the knob only. Draw back an amount of air into the syringe that is equal to the dose of modified insulin to be withdrawn.	
⎯	⎯	⎯	13. Hold the modified vial on a flat surface. Pierce the rubber stopper in the center with the needle tip and inject the measured air into the space above the solution. Do not inject air into the solution. Withdraw the needle.	
⎯	⎯	⎯	14. Draw back an amount of air into the syringe that is equal to the dose of unmodified insulin to be withdrawn.	

Excellent	Satisfactory	Needs Practice	

SKILL 29-4
Mixing Medications From Two Vials in One Syringe *(Continued)*

Comments

_____ _____ _____ 15. Hold the unmodified vial on a flat surface. Pierce the rubber stopper in the center with the needle tip and inject the measured air into the space above the solution. Do not inject air into the solution. Keep the needle in the vial.

_____ _____ _____ 16. Invert vial of unmodified insulin. Hold the vial in one hand and use the other to withdraw the medication. Touch the plunger at the knob only. *Draw up the prescribed amount of medication while holding the syringe at eye level and vertically.* Turn the vial over and then remove needle from vial.

_____ _____ _____ 17. Check that there are no air bubbles in the syringe.

_____ _____ _____ 18. *Check the amount of medication in the syringe with the medication dose and discard any surplus.*

_____ _____ _____ 19. *Recheck the vial label with the CMAR/MAR.*

_____ _____ _____ 20. Calculate the endpoint on the syringe for the combined insulin amount by adding the number of units for each dose together.

_____ _____ _____ 21. Insert the needle into the modified vial and invert it, taking care not to push the plunger and inject medication from the syringe into the vial. Invert vial of modified insulin. Hold the vial in one hand and use the other to withdraw the medication. Touch the plunger at the knob only. *Draw up the prescribed amount of medication while holding the syringe at eye level and vertically. Take care to only withdraw the prescribed amount.* Turn the vial over and then remove needle from vial. Carefully recap the needle. Carefully replace the cap over the needle.

_____ _____ _____ 22. *Check the amount of medication in the syringe with the medication dose.*

_____ _____ _____ 23. *Recheck the vial label with the CMAR/MAR.*

_____ _____ _____ 24. *Label the vials with the date and time opened, and store the vials containing the remaining medication according to facility policy.*

_____ _____ _____ 25. Lock medication cart before leaving it.

_____ _____ _____ 26. Perform hand hygiene.

_____ _____ _____ 27. Proceed with administration, based on prescribed route.

Skill Checklists for Fundamentals of Nursing:
The Art and Science of Nursing Care, 7th edition

Name _____ Date _____

Unit _____ Position _____

Instructor/Evaluator: _____ Position _____

Excellent	Satisfactory	Needs Practice	SKILL 29-5 **Administering an Intradermal Injection**	Comments
			Goal: Medication is safely injected intradermally causing a wheal to appear at the site of the injection.	
⎯	⎯	⎯	1. Gather equipment. Check each medication order against the original order in the medical record according to facility policy. Clarify any inconsistencies. Check the patient's chart for allergies.	
⎯	⎯	⎯	2. Know the actions, special nursing considerations, safe dose ranges, purpose of administration, and adverse effects of the medications to be administered. Consider the appropriateness of the medication for this patient.	
⎯	⎯	⎯	3. Perform hand hygiene.	
⎯	⎯	⎯	4. Move the medication cart to the outside of the patient's room or prepare for administration in the medication area.	
⎯	⎯	⎯	5. Unlock the medication cart or drawer. Enter pass code and scan employee identification, if required.	
⎯	⎯	⎯	6. *Prepare medications for one patient at a time.*	
⎯	⎯	⎯	7. Read the CMAR/MAR and select the proper medication from the patient's medication drawer or unit stock.	
⎯	⎯	⎯	8. Compare the label with the CMAR/MAR. Check expiration dates and perform calculations, if necessary. Scan the bar code on the package, if required.	
⎯	⎯	⎯	9. If necessary, withdraw medication from an ampule or vial, as described in Skills 29-2 and 29-3.	
⎯	⎯	⎯	10. *When all medications for one patient have been prepared, recheck the label with the CMAR/MAR before taking them to the patient.*	
⎯	⎯	⎯	11. Lock the medication cart before leaving it.	
⎯	⎯	⎯	12. Transport medications to the patient's bedside carefully, and keep the medications in sight at all times.	
⎯	⎯	⎯	13. *Ensure that the patient receives the medications at the correct time.*	
⎯	⎯	⎯	14. Perform hand hygiene and put on PPE, if indicated.	
⎯	⎯	⎯	15. Identify the patient. Usually, the patient should be identified using two methods. Compare information with the CMAR or MAR.	

Administering an Intradermal Injection (Continued)

Excellent	Satisfactory	Needs Practice		Comments
——	——	——	a. Check the name and identification number on the patient's identification band.	
——	——	——	b. Ask the patient to state his or her name and birth date, based on facility policy.	
——	——	——	c. If the patient cannot identify him- or herself, verify the patient's identification with a staff member who knows the patient for the second source.	
——	——	——	16. Close the door to the room or pull the bedside curtain.	
——	——	——	17. Complete necessary assessments before administering medications. Check allergy bracelet or ask the patient about allergies. Explain the purpose and action of the medication to the patient.	
——	——	——	18. Scan the patient's bar code on the identification band, if required.	
——	——	——	19. Put on clean gloves.	
——	——	——	20. Select an appropriate administration site. Assist the patient to the appropriate position for the site chosen. Drape as needed to expose only area of site to be used.	
——	——	——	21. Cleanse the site with an antimicrobial swab while wiping with a firm, circular motion and moving outward from the injection site. Allow the skin to dry.	
——	——	——	22. Remove the needle cap with the nondominant hand by pulling it straight off.	
——	——	——	23. Use the nondominant hand to spread the skin taut over the injection site.	
——	——	——	24. Hold the syringe in the dominant hand, between the thumb and forefinger with the bevel of the needle up.	
——	——	——	25. Hold the syringe at a 5- to 15- degree angle from the site. *Place the needle almost flat against the patient's skin, bevel side up, and insert the needle into the skin. Insert the needle only about ⅛″ with entire bevel under the skin.*	
——	——	——	26. Once the needle is in place, steady the lower end of the syringe. Slide your dominant hand to the end of the plunger.	
——	——	——	27. Slowly inject the agent while watching for a small wheal or blister to appear.	
——	——	——	28. Withdraw the needle quickly at the same angle that it was inserted. Do not recap the used needle. Engage the safety shield or needle guard.	

Excellent	Satisfactory	Needs Practice	SKILL 29-5 **Administering an Intradermal Injection** *(Continued)*	
				Comments
——	——	——	29. *Do not massage the area after removing needle. Tell patient not to rub or scratch the site. If necessary, gently blot the site with a dry gauze square. Do not apply pressure or rub the site.*	
——	——	——	30. Assist the patient to a position of comfort.	
——	——	——	31. Discard the needle and syringe in the appropriate receptacle.	
——	——	——	32. Remove gloves and additional PPE, if used. Perform hand hygiene.	
——	——	——	33. Document the administration of the medication immediately after administration.	
——	——	——	34. Evaluate patient's response to medication within appropriate time frame.	
——	——	——	35. Observe the area for signs of a reaction at determined intervals after administration. Inform the patient of the need for inspection.	

Skill Checklists for Fundamentals of Nursing:
The Art and Science of Nursing Care, 7th edition

Name _____   Date _____

Unit _____   Position _____

Instructor/Evaluator: _____   Position _____

Excellent	Satisfactory	Needs Practice	SKILL 29-6 **Administering a Subcutaneous Injection**	Comments
			Goal: The patient safely receives medication via the subcutaneous route.	
___	___	___	1. Gather equipment. Check each medication order against the original order in the medical record, according to facility policy. Clarify any inconsistencies. Check the patient's chart for allergies.	
___	___	___	2. Know the actions, special nursing considerations, safe dose ranges, purpose of administration, and adverse effects of the medications to be administered. Consider the appropriateness of the medication for this patient.	
___	___	___	3. Perform hand hygiene.	
___	___	___	4. Move the medication cart to the outside of the patient's room or prepare for administration in the medication area.	
___	___	___	5. Unlock the medication cart or drawer. Enter pass code and scan employee identification, if required.	
___	___	___	6. *Prepare medications for one patient at a time.*	
___	___	___	7. Read the CMAR/MAR and select the proper medication from the patient's medication drawer or unit stock.	
___	___	___	8. Compare the label with the CMAR/MAR. Check expiration dates and perform calculations, if necessary. Scan the bar code on the package, if required.	
___	___	___	9. If necessary, withdraw medication from an ampule or vial as described in Skills 29-2 and 29-3.	
___	___	___	10. *When all medications for one patient have been prepared, recheck the label with the MAR before taking them to the patient.*	
___	___	___	11. Lock the medication cart before leaving it.	
___	___	___	12. Transport medications to the patient's bedside carefully, and keep the medications in sight at all times.	
___	___	___	13. *Ensure that the patient receives the medications at the correct time.*	
___	___	___	14. Perform hand hygiene and put on PPE, if indicated.	
___	___	___	15. Identify the patient. Usually, the patient should be identified using two methods. Compare information with the CMAR or MAR.	

SKILL 29-6

Administering a Subcutaneous Injection *(Continued)*

Excellent	Satisfactory	Needs Practice		Comments
——	——	——	a. Check the name and identification number on the patient's identification band.	
——	——	——	b. Ask the patient to state his or her name and birth date, based on facility policy.	
——	——	——	c. If the patient cannot identify him- or herself, verify the patient's identification with a staff member who knows the patient for the second source.	
——	——	——	16. Close the door to the room or pull the bedside curtain.	
——	——	——	17. Complete necessary assessments before administering medications. Check the patient's allergy bracelet or ask the patient about allergies. Explain the purpose and action of the medication to the patient.	
——	——	——	18. Scan the patient's bar code on the identification band, if required.	
——	——	——	19. Put on clean gloves.	
——	——	——	20. Select an appropriate administration site.	
——	——	——	21. Assist the patient to the appropriate position for the site chosen. Drape as needed to expose only area of site to be used.	
——	——	——	22. Identify the appropriate landmarks for the site chosen.	
——	——	——	23. Cleanse the area around the injection site with an antimicrobial swab. Use a firm, circular motion while moving outward from the injection site. Allow area to dry.	
——	——	——	24. Remove the needle cap with the nondominant hand, pulling it straight off.	
——	——	——	25. Grasp and bunch the area surrounding the injection site or spread the skin taut at the site.	
——	——	——	26. ***Hold the syringe in the dominant hand between the thumb and forefinger. Inject the needle quickly at a 45- to 90-degree angle.***	
——	——	——	27. After the needle is in place, release the tissue. If you have a large skin fold pinched up, ensure that the needle stays in place as the skin is released. Immediately move your nondominant hand to steady the lower end of the syringe. Slide your dominant hand to the end of the plunger. Avoid moving the syringe.	
——	——	——	28. Inject the medication slowly (at a rate of 10 seconds per milliliter).	
——	——	——	29. Withdraw the needle quickly at the same angle at which it was inserted, while supporting the surrounding tissue with your nondominant hand.	

SKILL 29-6

Administering a Subcutaneous Injection *(Continued)*

Excellent	Satisfactory	Needs Practice		Comments
———	———	———	30. Using a gauze square, apply gentle pressure to the site after the needle is withdrawn. Do not massage the site.	
———	———	———	31. Do not recap the used needle. Engage the safety shield or needle guard. Discard the needle and syringe in the appropriate receptacle.	
———	———	———	32. Assist the patient to a position of comfort.	
———	———	———	33. Remove gloves and additional PPE, if used. Perform hand hygiene.	
———	———	———	34. Document the administration of the medication immediately after administration.	
———	———	———	35. Evaluate the response of the patient to the medication within an appropriate time frame for the particular medication.	

Skill Checklists for Fundamentals of Nursing:
The Art and Science of Nursing Care, 7th edition

Name _____ Date _____

Unit _____ Position _____

Instructor/Evaluator: _____ Position _____

SKILL 29-7
Administering an Intramuscular Injection

Goal: The patient safely receives the medication via the intramuscular route using a Z-track method.

Excellent	Satisfactory	Needs Practice		Comments
___	___	___	1. Gather equipment. Check each medication order against the original order in the medical record according to facility policy. Clarify any inconsistencies. Check the patient's chart for allergies.	
___	___	___	2. Know the actions, special nursing considerations, safe dose ranges, purpose of administration, and adverse effects of the medications to be administered. Consider the appropriateness of the medication for this patient.	
___	___	___	3. Perform hand hygiene.	
___	___	___	4. Move the medication cart to the outside of the patient's room or prepare for administration in the medication area.	
___	___	___	5. Unlock the medication cart or drawer. Enter pass code and scan employee identification, if required.	
___	___	___	6. *Prepare medications for one patient at a time.*	
___	___	___	7. Read the CMAR/MAR and select the proper medication from the patient's medication drawer or unit stock.	
___	___	___	8. Compare the label with the CMAR/MAR. Check expiration dates and perform calculations, if necessary. Scan the bar code on the package, if required.	
___	___	___	9. If necessary, withdraw medication from an ampule or vial, as described in Skills 29-2 and 29-3.	
___	___	___	10. *When all medications for one patient have been prepared, recheck the label with the MAR before taking them to the patient.*	
___	___	___	11. Lock the medication cart before leaving it.	
___	___	___	12. Transport medications to the patient's bedside carefully, and keep the medications in sight at all times.	
___	___	___	13. *Ensure that the patient receives the medications at the correct time.*	
___	___	___	14. Perform hand hygiene and put on PPE, if indicated.	
___	___	___	15. Identify the patient. Usually, the patient should be identified using two methods. Compare information with the CMAR or MAR.	

Excellent	Satisfactory	Needs Practice	SKILL 29-7 **Administering an Intramuscular Injection** *(Continued)*	
				Comments
——	——	——	a. Check the name and identification number on the patient's identification band.	
——	——	——	b. Ask the patient to state his or her name and birth date, based on facility policy.	
——	——	——	c. If the patient cannot identify him- or herself, verify the patient's identification with a staff member who knows the patient for the second source.	
——	——	——	16. Close the door to the room or pull the bedside curtain.	
——	——	——	17. Complete necessary assessments before administering medications. Check the patient's allergy bracelet or ask the patient about allergies. Explain the purpose and action of the medication to the patient.	
——	——	——	18. Scan the patient's bar code on the identification band, if required.	
——	——	——	19. Put on clean gloves.	
——	——	——	20. Select an appropriate administration site.	
——	——	——	21. Assist the patient to the appropriate position for the site chosen. Drape as needed to expose only the area of site being used.	
——	——	——	22. *Identify the appropriate landmarks for the site chosen.*	
——	——	——	23. Cleanse the area around the injection site with an antimicrobial swab. Use a firm, circular motion while moving outward from the injection site. Allow area to dry.	
——	——	——	24. Remove the needle cap by pulling it straight off. Hold the syringe in your dominant hand between the thumb and forefinger.	
——	——	——	25. Displace the skin in a Z-track manner by pulling the skin down or to one side about 1″ (2.5 cm) with your nondominant hand and hold the skin and tissue in this position.	
——	——	——	26. Quickly dart the needle into the tissue so that the needle is perpendicular to the patient's body. This should ensure that it is given using an angle of injection between 72 and 90 degrees.	
——	——	——	27. As soon as the needle is in place, use the thumb and forefinger of your nondominant hand to hold the lower end of the syringe. Slide your dominant hand to the end of the plunger. Inject the solution slowly (10 seconds per milliliter of medication).	
——	——	——	28. Once the medication has been instilled, wait 10 seconds before withdrawing the needle.	

Excellent	Satisfactory	Needs Practice	SKILL 29-7 **Administering an Intramuscular Injection** *(Continued)*	Comments
——	——	——	29. Withdraw the needle smoothly and steadily at the same angle at which it was inserted, supporting tissue around the injection site with your nondominant hand.	
——	——	——	30. *Apply gentle pressure at the site with a dry gauze.* Do not massage the site.	
——	——	——	31. Do not recap the used needle. Engage the safety shield or needle guard, if present. Discard the needle and syringe in the appropriate receptacle.	
——	——	——	32. Assist the patient to a position of comfort.	
——	——	——	33. Remove gloves and additional PPE, if used. Perform hand hygiene.	
——	——	——	34. Document the administration of the medication immediately after administration.	
——	——	——	35. Evaluate patient's response to medication within an appropriate time frame. Assess site, if possible, within 2 to 4 hours after administration.	

Skill Checklists for Fundamentals of Nursing:
The Art and Science of Nursing Care, 7th edition

Name _____ Date _____

Unit _____ Position _____

Instructor/Evaluator: _____ Position _____

Excellent	Satisfactory	Needs Practice	SKILL 29-8 **Administering Medications by Intravenous Bolus or Push Through an Intravenous Infusion** **Goal:** The prescribed medication is given safely to the patient via the intravenous route.	Comments
____	____	____	1. Gather equipment. Check medication order against the original order in the medical record, according to facility policy. Clarify any inconsistencies. Check the patient's chart for allergies. Verify the compatibility of the medication and IV fluid. Check a drug resource to clarify whether the medication needs to be diluted before administration. Check the infusion rate.	
____	____	____	2. Know the actions, special nursing considerations, safe dose ranges, purpose of administration, and adverse effects of the medications to be administered. Consider the appropriateness of the medication for this patient.	
____	____	____	3. Perform hand hygiene.	
____	____	____	4. Move the medication cart to the outside of the patient's room or prepare for administration in the medication area.	
____	____	____	5. Unlock the medication cart or drawer. Enter pass code and scan employee identification, if required.	
____	____	____	6. *Prepare medication for one patient at a time.*	
____	____	____	7. Read the CMAR/MAR and select the proper medication from the patient's medication drawer or unit stock.	
____	____	____	8. Compare the label with the CMAR/MAR. Check expiration dates and perform calculations, if necessary. Scan the bar code on the package, if required.	
____	____	____	9. If necessary, withdraw medication from an ampule or vial, as described in Skills 29-2 and 29-3.	
____	____	____	10. *Recheck the label with the MAR before taking it to the patient.*	
____	____	____	11. Lock the medication cart before leaving it.	
____	____	____	12. Transport medications and equipment to the patient's bedside carefully, and keep the medications in sight at all times.	
____	____	____	13. *Ensure that the patient receives the medications at the correct time.*	
____	____	____	14. Perform hand hygiene and put on PPE, if indicated.	
____	____	____	15. Identify the patient. Usually, the patient should be identified using two methods. Compare information with the CMAR or MAR.	

Excellent	Satisfactory	Needs Practice		

SKILL 29-8

Administering Medications by Intravenous Bolus or Push Through an Intravenous Infusion *(Continued)*

				Comments

——	——	——	a. Check the name and identification number on the patient's identification band.	
——	——	——	b. Ask the patient to state his or her name and birth date, based on facility policy.	
——	——	——	c. If the patient cannot identify him- or herself, verify the patient's identification with a staff member who knows the patient for the second source.	
——	——	——	16. Close the door to the room or pull the bedside curtain.	
——	——	——	17. Complete necessary assessments before administering medications. Check the patient's allergy bracelet or ask the patient about allergies. Explain the purpose and action of the medication to the patient.	
——	——	——	18. Scan the patient's bar code on the identification band, if required.	
——	——	——	19. *Assess IV site for presence of inflammation or infiltration.*	
——	——	——	20. If IV infusion is being administered via an infusion pump, pause the pump.	
——	——	——	21. Put on clean gloves.	
——	——	——	22. Select injection port on tubing that is closest to venipuncture site. Clean port with antimicrobial swab.	
——	——	——	23. Uncap syringe. Steady port with your nondominant hand while inserting syringe into center of port.	
——	——	——	24. Move your nondominant hand to the section of IV tubing just above the injection port. Fold the tubing between your fingers.	
——	——	——	25. Pull back slightly on plunger just until blood appears in tubing.	
——	——	——	26. *Inject the medication at the recommended rate.*	
——	——	——	27. Release the tubing. Remove the syringe. Do not recap the used needle, if used. Engage the safety shield or needle guard, if present. Release the tubing and allow the IV fluid to flow. Discard the needle and syringe in the appropriate receptacle.	
——	——	——	28. Check IV fluid infusion rate. Restart infusion pump, if appropriate.	
——	——	——	29. Remove gloves and additional PPE, if used. Perform hand hygiene.	
——	——	——	30. Document the administration of the medication immediately after administration.	
——	——	——	31. Evaluate patient's response to medication within appropriate time frame.	

Skill Checklists for Fundamentals of Nursing:
The Art and Science of Nursing Care, 7th edition

Name _____   Date _____

Unit _____   Position _____

Instructor/Evaluator: _____   Position _____

SKILL 29-9

Administering a Piggyback Intermittent Intravenous Infusion of Medication

Goal: The medication is delivered safely to the patient via the intravenous route using sterile technique.

Excellent	Satisfactory	Needs Practice		Comments
___	___	___	1. Gather equipment. Check each medication order against the original order in the medical record, according to facility policy. Clarify any inconsistencies. Check the patient's chart for allergies.	
___	___	___	2. Know the actions, special nursing considerations, safe dose ranges, purpose of administration, and adverse effects of the medications to be administered. Consider the appropriateness of the medication for this patient.	
___	___	___	3. Perform hand hygiene.	
___	___	___	4. Move the medication cart to the outside of the patient's room or prepare for administration in the medication area.	
___	___	___	5. Unlock the medication cart or drawer. Enter pass code and scan employee identification, if required.	
___	___	___	6. *Prepare medications for one patient at a time.*	
___	___	___	7. Read the CMAR/MAR and select the proper medication from the patient's medication drawer or unit stock.	
___	___	___	8. Compare the label with the CMAR/MAR. Check expiration dates. Confirm the prescribed or appropriate infusion rate. Calculate the drip rate if using gravity system. Scan the bar code on the package, if required.	
___	___	___	9. *When all medications for one patient have been prepared, recheck the label with the MAR before taking them to the patient.*	
___	___	___	10. Lock the medication cart before leaving it.	
___	___	___	11. Transport medications to the patient's bedside carefully, and keep the medications in sight at all times.	
___	___	___	12. *Ensure that the patient receives the medications at the correct time.*	
___	___	___	13. Perform hand hygiene and put on PPE, if indicated.	
___	___	___	14. Identify the patient. Usually, the patient should be identified using two methods. Compare information with the CMAR or MAR.	

SKILL 29-9

Administering a Piggyback Intermittent Intravenous Infusion of Medication *(Continued)*

Excellent	Satisfactory	Needs Practice		Comments
—	—	—	a. Check the name and identification number on the patient's identification band.	
—	—	—	b. Ask the patient to state his or her name and birth date, based on facility policy.	
—	—	—	c. If the patient cannot identify him- or herself, verify the patient's identification with a staff member who knows the patient for the second source.	
—	—	—	15. Close the door to the room or pull the bedside curtain.	
—	—	—	16. Complete necessary assessments before administering medications. Check the patient's allergy bracelet or ask the patient about allergies. Explain the purpose and action of the medication to the patient.	
—	—	—	17. Scan the patient's bar code on the identification band, if required.	
—	—	—	18. Assess the IV site for the presence of inflammation or infiltration.	
—	—	—	19. Close the clamp on the short secondary infusion tubing. Using aseptic technique, remove the cap on the tubing spike and the cap on the port of the medication container, taking care to avoid contaminating either end.	
—	—	—	20. Attach infusion tubing to the medication container by inserting the tubing spike into the port with a firm push and twisting motion, taking care to avoid contaminating either end.	
—	—	—	21. Hang piggyback container on IV pole, positioning it higher than primary IV according to manufacturer's recommendations. Use metal or plastic hook to lower primary IV fluid container.	
—	—	—	22. Place label on tubing with appropriate date.	
—	—	—	23. Squeeze drip chamber on tubing and release. Fill to the line or about half full. Open clamp and prime tubing. Close clamp. Place needleless connector on the end of the tubing, using sterile technique, if required.	
—	—	—	24. Use an antimicrobial swab to clean the access port or stopcock above the roller clamp on the primary IV infusion tubing.	
—	—	—	25. Connect piggyback setup to the access port or stopcock. If using, turn the stopcock to the open position.	

Administering a Piggyback Intermittent Intravenous Infusion of Medication *(Continued)*

Excellent	Satisfactory	Needs Practice		Comments
⎯⎯	⎯⎯	⎯⎯	26. Open clamp on the secondary tubing. Set rate for secondary infusion on infusion pump and begin infusion. If using gravity infusion, use the roller clamp on the primary infusion tubing to regulate flow at prescribed delivery rate. Monitor medication infusion at periodic intervals.	
⎯⎯	⎯⎯	⎯⎯	27. Clamp tubing on piggyback set when solution is infused. Follow facility policy regarding disposal of equipment.	
⎯⎯	⎯⎯	⎯⎯	28. Replace primary IV fluid container to original height. ***Check primary infusion rate on infusion pump. If using gravity infusion, readjust flow rate of primary IV.***	
⎯⎯	⎯⎯	⎯⎯	29. Remove PPE, if used. Perform hand hygiene.	
⎯⎯	⎯⎯	⎯⎯	30. Document the administration of the medication immediately after administration.	
⎯⎯	⎯⎯	⎯⎯	31. Evaluate patient's response to medication within appropriate time frame. Monitor IV site at periodic intervals.	

Skill Checklists for Fundamentals of Nursing:
The Art and Science of Nursing Care, 7th edition

Name _____ Date _____

Unit _____ Position _____

Instructor/Evaluator: _____ Position _____

Excellent	Satisfactory	Needs Practice	SKILL 29-10 **Introducing Drugs Through a Medication or Drug-Infusion Lock (Intermittent Peripheral Venous Access Device) Using the Saline Flush**	Comments
			Goal: The medication is delivered safely to the patient via the intravenous route using sterile technique.	
——	——	——	1. Gather equipment. Check the medication order against the original order in the medical record, according to agency policy. Clarify any inconsistencies. Check the patient's chart for allergies. Check a drug resource to clarify whether medication needs to be diluted before administration. Verify the recommended infusion rate.	
——	——	——	2. Know the actions, special nursing considerations, safe dose ranges, purpose of administration, and adverse effects of the medications to be administered. Consider the appropriateness of the medication for this patient.	
——	——	——	3. Perform hand hygiene.	
——	——	——	4. Move the medication cart to the outside of the patient's room or prepare for administration in the medication area.	
——	——	——	5. Unlock the medication cart or drawer. Enter pass code and scan employee identification, if required.	
——	——	——	6. *Prepare medication for one patient at a time.*	
——	——	——	7. Read the CMAR/MAR and select the proper medication from the patient's medication drawer or unit stock.	
——	——	——	8. Compare the label with the CMAR/MAR. Check expiration dates and perform calculations, if necessary. Scan the bar code on the package, if required.	
——	——	——	9. If necessary, withdraw medication from an ampule or vial, as described in Skills 29-2 and 29-3.	
——	——	——	10. *When all medications for one patient have been prepared, recheck the label with the MAR before taking them to the patient.*	
——	——	——	11. Lock the medication cart before leaving it.	
——	——	——	12. Transport medications and equipment to the patient's bedside carefully, and keep the medications in sight at all times.	
——	——	——	13. *Ensure that the patient receives the medications at the correct time.*	
——	——	——	14. Perform hand hygiene and put on PPE, if indicated.	

Introducing Drugs Through a Medication or Drug-Infusion Lock (Intermittent Peripheral Venous Access Device) Using the Saline Flush *(Continued)*

Excellent	Satisfactory	Needs Practice		Comments
___	___	___	15. Identify the patient. Usually, the patient should be identified using two methods. Compare information with the MAR or CMAR.	
___	___	___	a. Check the name and identification number on the patient's identification band.	
___	___	___	b. Ask the patient to state his or her name and birth date, based on facility policy.	
___	___	___	c. If the patient cannot identify him- or herself, verify the patient's identification with a staff member who knows the patient for the second source.	
___	___	___	16. Close the door to the room or pull the bedside curtain.	
___	___	___	17. Complete necessary assessments before administering medications. Check the patient's allergy bracelet or ask the patient about allergies. Explain the purpose and action of the medication to the patient.	
___	___	___	18. Scan the patient's bar code on the identification band, if required.	
___	___	___	19. Assess IV site for presence of inflammation or infiltration.	
___	___	___	20. Put on clean gloves.	
___	___	___	21. Clean the access port of the medication lock with antimicrobial swab.	
___	___	___	22. Stabilize the port with your nondominant hand and insert the syringe, or needleless access device, of normal saline into the access port.	
___	___	___	23. Release the clamp on the extension tubing of the medication lock. Aspirate gently and check for blood return.	
___	___	___	24. Gently flush with normal saline by pushing slowly on the syringe plunger. Observe the insertion site while inserting the saline. Remove syringe.	
___	___	___	25. Insert syringe, or needleless access device, with medication into the port and gently inject medication, using a watch to verify correct administration rate. ***Do not force the injection if resistance is felt.***	

SKILL 29-10

Introducing Drugs Through a Medication or Drug-Infusion Lock (Intermittent Peripheral Venous Access Device) Using the Saline Flush *(Continued)*

Excellent	Satisfactory	Needs Practice		Comments
――	――	――	26. Remove the medication syringe from the port. Stabilize the port with your nondominant hand and insert the syringe, or needleless access device, of normal saline into the port. Gently flush with normal saline by pushing slowly on the syringe plunger. ***If medication lock is capped with positive pressure valve/device, remove syringe, and then clamp the IV tubing.*** Alternately, to gain positive pressure if positive pressure valve/device is not present, clamp the IV tubing as you are still flushing the last of the saline into the medication lock. Remove syringe.	
――	――	――	27. Discard the syringe in the appropriate receptacle.	
――	――	――	28. Remove PPE, if used. Perform hand hygiene.	
――	――	――	29. Document the administration of the medication immediately after administration.	
――	――	――	30. Evaluate the patient's response to medication within appropriate time frame.	
――	――	――	31. Check the medication lock site at least every 8 hours or according to facility policy.	

Name _____   Date _____

Unit _____   Position _____

Instructor/Evaluator: _____   Position _____

SKILL 30-1

Providing Preoperative Patient Care: Hospitalized Patient

Goal: The patient will be prepared physically and psychologically to proceed to surgery.

Excellent	Satisfactory	Needs Practice		Comments
——	——	——	1. Check the patient's chart for the type of surgery and review the medical orders. Review the nursing database, history, and physical examination. Check that the baseline data are recorded; report those that are abnormal.	
——	——	——	2. ***Check that diagnostic testing has been completed and results are available; identify and report abnormal results.***	
——	——	——	3. Gather the necessary supplies and bring to the bedside stand or overbed table.	
——	——	——	4. Perform hand hygiene and put on PPE, if indicated.	
——	——	——	5. Identify the patient.	
——	——	——	6. Close curtains around bed and close door to room if possible. Explain what you are going to do and why you are going to do it to the patient.	
——	——	——	7. Explore the psychological needs of the patient related to the surgery as well as the family.	
——	——	——	a. Establish the therapeutic relationship, encouraging the patient to verbalize concerns or fears.	
——	——	——	b. Use active learning skills, answering questions and clarifying any misinformation.	
——	——	——	c. Use touch, as appropriate, to convey genuine empathy.	
——	——	——	d. Offer to contact spiritual counselor (priest, minister, rabbi) to meet spiritual needs.	
——	——	——	8. ***Identify learning needs of patient and family.*** Ensure that the informed consent of the patient for the surgery has been signed, witnessed, and dated. Inquire if the patient has any questions regarding the surgical procedure. Check the patient's record to determine if an advance directive has been completed. If an advance directive has not been completed, discuss with the patient the possibility of completing as appropriate. If patient has had surgery before, ask about this experience.	
——	——	——	9. Provide teaching about deep-breathing exercises. (See Guidelines for Nursing Care 30-1 for specific technique.)	

Excellent	Satisfactory	Needs Practice		
			SKILL 30-1 **Providing Preoperative Patient Care: Hospitalized Patient** *(Continued)*	
				Comments
——	——	——	10. Provide teaching regarding coughing and splinting (providing support to the incision). (See Guidelines for Nursing Care 30-2 for specific technique.)	
——	——	——	11. Provide teaching regarding incentive spirometer. (See Chapter 39, Guidelines for Nursing Care 39-1.)	
——	——	——	12. Provide teaching regarding leg exercises (as appropriate).	
——	——	——	13. Assist the patient in putting on antiembolism stockings and demonstrate how the pneumatic compression device operates. (Refer to Chapter 33 for specific information.)	
——	——	——	14. Provide teaching regarding turning in the bed.	
——	——	——	a. Instruct the patient to use a pillow or bath blanket to splint where the incision will be. Ask the patient to raise his or her left knee and reach across to grasp the right side rail of the bed when he/she is turning toward his or her right side. If patient is turning to his or her left side, he or she will bend the right knee and grasp the left side rail.	
——	——	——	b. When turning the patient onto his or her right side, ask the patient to push with bent left leg and pull on the right side rail. Explain to patient that the nurse will place a pillow behind his/her back to provide support, and that the call bell will be placed within easy reach.	
——	——	——	c. Explain to the patient that position change is recommended every 2 hours.	
——	——	——	15. Provide teaching about pain management.	
——	——	——	a. Discuss past experiences with pain and interventions that the patient has used to reduce pain.	
——	——	——	b. Discuss the availability of analgesic medication postoperatively.	
——	——	——	c. Discuss the use of patient controlled analgesia (PCA), as appropriate. (Refer to Chapter 35.)	
——	——	——	d. Explore the use of other alternative and nonpharmacologic methods to reduce pain such as position change, massage, relaxation/diversion, guided imagery, and meditation.	
——	——	——	16. Review equipment that may be used.	
——	——	——	a. Show the patient various equipment such as IV pumps, electronic blood pressure cuff, tubes, and surgical drains.	
——	——	——	17. Provide skin preparation.	
——	——	——	a. *Ask the patient to bathe or shower with the antiseptic solution. Remind the patient to clean the surgical site.*	

Excellent	Satisfactory	Needs Practice	SKILL 30-1 **Providing Preoperative Patient Care:** **Hospitalized Patient** *(Continued)*	
				Comments
——	——	——	18. Provide teaching about following dietary/fluid restrictions.	
——	——	——	a. *Explain to the patient that both food and fluid will be restricted before surgery to ensure that the stomach contains a minimal amount of gastric secretions. This restriction is important to reduce the risk of aspiration. Emphasize to the patient the importance of avoiding food and fluids during the prescribed time period, since failure to adhere may necessitate cancellation of the surgery.*	
——	——	——	19. Provide intestinal preparation, as appropriate. In certain situations, the bowel will need to be prepared through the administering of enemas or laxatives to evacuate the bowel and to reduce the intestinal bacteria.	
——	——	——	a. *As needed, provide explanation of the purpose of enemas or laxatives before surgery. If patient will be administering an enema, clarify the steps as needed.*	
——	——	——	20. *Check administration of regularly scheduled medications.* Review with patient routine medications, over-the-counter medications, and herbal supplements that are taken regularly. Check the physician's orders and review with patient which meds he/she will be permitted to take the day of surgery.	
——	——	——	21. Remove PPE, if used. Perform hand hygiene.	

Skill Checklists for Fundamentals of Nursing:
The Art and Science of Nursing Care, 7th edition

Name _____ Date _____

Unit _____ Position _____

Instructor/Evaluator: _____ Position _____

Excellent	Satisfactory	Needs Practice	SKILL 30-2 **Providing Postoperative Care** **When Patient Returns to Room** **Goal:** The patient will recover from the surgery with postoperative risks minimized by frequent assessments.	Comments
⎯⎯	⎯⎯	⎯⎯	1. When patient returns from the PACU, obtain a report from the PACU nurse and review the operating room and PACU data.	
⎯⎯	⎯⎯	⎯⎯	2. Perform hand hygiene and put on PPE, if indicated.	
⎯⎯	⎯⎯	⎯⎯	3. Identify the patient.	
⎯⎯	⎯⎯	⎯⎯	4. Close curtains around bed and close door to room if possible. Explain what you are going to do and why you are going to do it to the patient.	
⎯⎯	⎯⎯	⎯⎯	5. *Place patient in safe position (semi- or high Fowler's or side-lying). Note level of consciousness.*	
⎯⎯	⎯⎯	⎯⎯	6. *Obtain vital signs. Monitor and record vital signs frequently.* Assessment order may vary, but usual frequency includes taking vital signs every 15 minutes the first hour, every 30 minutes the next 2 hours, every hour for 4 hours, and finally every 4 hours.	
⎯⎯	⎯⎯	⎯⎯	7. Assess the patient's respiratory status. (Refer to Chapter 25.) Measure the patient's oxygen saturation level.	
⎯⎯	⎯⎯	⎯⎯	8. Assess the patient's cardiovascular status. (Refer to Chapter 25.)	
⎯⎯	⎯⎯	⎯⎯	9. Assess the patient's neurovascular status, based on the type of surgery performed. (Refer to Chapter 25.)	
⎯⎯	⎯⎯	⎯⎯	10. Provide for warmth, using heated or extra blankets as necessary. Assess skin color and condition.	
⎯⎯	⎯⎯	⎯⎯	11. Check dressings for color, odor, presence of drains, and amount of drainage. Mark the drainage on the dressing by circling the amount and include the time. Turn the patient to visually assess under the patient for bleeding from the surgical site.	
⎯⎯	⎯⎯	⎯⎯	12. Verify that all tubes and drains are patent and equipment is operative; note amount of drainage in collection device. If an indwelling urinary (Foley) catheter is in place, note urinary output.	
⎯⎯	⎯⎯	⎯⎯	13. Verify and maintain IV infusion at correct rate.	

Excellent	Satisfactory	Needs Practice	SKILL 30-2 **Providing Postoperative Care When Patient Returns to Room** *(Continued)*	
				Comments
——	——	——	14. Assess for and relieve pain by administering medications ordered by physician. If patient has been instructed in use of PCA for pain management, review use. Check record to verify if analgesic medication was administered in the PACU.	
——	——	——	15. Provide for a safe environment. Keep bed in low position with side rails up, based on facility policy. Have call bell within patient's reach.	
——	——	——	16. Remove PPE, if used. Perform hand hygiene.	
			Ongoing Care	
——	——	——	17. Promote optimal respiratory function.	
——	——	——	a. Assess respiratory rate, depth, quality, color, and capillary refill. Ask if the patient is experiencing any difficulty breathing.	
——	——	——	b. Assist with coughing and deep-breathing exercises (Refer to Guidelines for Nursing Care 30-1 and 30-2).	
——	——	——	c. Assist with incentive spirometry.	
——	——	——	d. Assist with early ambulation.	
——	——	——	e. Provide frequent position change.	
——	——	——	f. Administer oxygen, as ordered.	
——	——	——	g. Monitor pulse oximetry.	
——	——	——	18. Promote optimal cardiovascular function:	
——	——	——	a. Assess apical rate, rhythm, and quality and compare to peripheral pulses, color, and blood pressure. Ask if the patient has any chest pains or shortness of breath.	
——	——	——	b. Provide frequent position changes.	
——	——	——	c. Assist with early ambulation.	
——	——	——	d. Apply antiembolism stockings or pneumatic compression devices, if ordered and not in place. If in place, assess for integrity.	
——	——	——	e. Provide leg and range-of-motion exercises if not contraindicated.	
——	——	——	19. Promote optimal neurologic function:	
——	——	——	a. Assess level of consciousness, motor, and sensation.	
——	——	——	b. Determine the level of orientation to person, place, and time.	
——	——	——	c. Test motor ability by asking the patient to move each extremity.	

Excellent	Satisfactory	Needs Practice		
			SKILL 30-2 **Providing Postoperative Care** **When Patient Returns to Room** *(Continued)*	
				Comments
——	——	——	d. Evaluate sensation by asking the patient if he or she can feel your touch on an extremity.	
——	——	——	20. Promote optimal renal and urinary function and fluid and electrolyte status. Assess intake and output, evaluate for urinary retention, and monitor serum electrolyte levels.	
——	——	——	a. Promote voiding by offering bedpan at regular intervals, noting the frequency, amount, and if any burning or urgency symptoms.	
——	——	——	b. Monitor urinary catheter drainage if present.	
——	——	——	c. Measure intake and output.	
——	——	——	21. Promote optimal gastrointestinal function and meet nutritional needs:	
——	——	——	a. Assess abdomen for distention and firmness. Ask if patient feels nauseated, any vomiting, and if passing flatus.	
——	——	——	b. Auscultate for bowel sounds.	
——	——	——	c. Assist with diet progression, encourage fluid intake, and monitor intake.	
——	——	——	d. Medicate for nausea and vomiting as ordered by physician.	
——	——	——	22. Promote optimal wound healing.	
——	——	——	a. Assess condition of wound for presence of drains and any drainage.	
——	——	——	b. Use surgical asepsis for dressing changes.	
——	——	——	c. Inspect all skin surfaces for beginning signs of pressure ulcer development and use pressure-relieving supports to minimize potential skin breakdown.	
——	——	——	23. Promote optimal comfort and relief from pain.	
——	——	——	a. Assess for pain (location and intensity using scale).	
——	——	——	b. Provide for rest and comfort; provide extra blankets as needed for warmth.	
——	——	——	c. Administer pain medications, as needed, or other nonpharmacologic methods.	
——	——	——	24. Promote optimal meeting of psychosocial needs:	
——	——	——	a. Provide emotional support to patient and family, as needed.	
——	——	——	b. Explain procedures and offer explanations regarding postoperative recovery as needed to both patient and family members.	

Skill Checklists for Fundamentals of Nursing:
The Art and Science of Nursing Care, 7th edition

Name _____   Date _____

Unit _____   Position _____

Instructor/Evaluator: _____   Position _____

SKILL 31-1

Giving a Bed Bath

Excellent	Satisfactory	Needs Practice		Comments
			Goal: The patient will vocalize feeling clean and fresh.	
——	——	——	1. Review chart for any limitations in physical activity.	
——	——	——	2. Bring necessary equipment to the bedside stand or overbed table.	
——	——	——	3. Perform hand hygiene and put on gloves and/or other PPE, if indicated.	
——	——	——	4. Identify the patient. Discuss procedure with patient and assess patient's ability to assist in the bathing process, as well as personal hygiene preferences.	
——	——	——	5. Close curtains around bed and close door to room if possible. Adjust the room temperature if necessary.	
——	——	——	6. Remove sequential compression devices and antiembolism stockings from lower extremities according to agency protocol.	
——	——	——	7. Offer patient bedpan or urinal.	
——	——	——	8. Remove gloves and perform hand hygiene.	
——	——	——	9. Adjust the bed to a comfortable working height; usually elbow height of the caregiver (VISN 8, 2009).	
——	——	——	10. Put on gloves. Lower side rail nearer to you and assist patient to side of bed where you will work. Have patient lie on his or her back.	
——	——	——	11. Loosen top covers and remove all except the top sheet. Place bath blanket over patient and then remove top sheet while patient holds bath blanket in place. If linen is to be reused, fold it over a chair. Place soiled linen in laundry bag. Take care to prevent linen from coming in contact with your clothing.	
——	——	——	12. Remove patient's gown and keep bath blanket in place. If patient has an IV line and is not wearing a gown with snap sleeves, remove gown from other arm first. *Lower the IV container and pass gown over the tubing and the container. Rehang the container and check the drip rate.*	

SKILL 31-1
Giving a Bed Bath *(Continued)*

Excellent	Satisfactory	Needs Practice		Comments
——	——	——	13. *Raise side rails.* Fill basin with a sufficient amount of comfortably warm water (110°–115°F). Add the skin cleanser, if appropriate, according to manufacturer's directions. Change as necessary throughout the bath. Lower side rail closer to you when you return to the bedside to begin the bath.	
——	——	——	14. Put on gloves, if necessary. Fold the washcloth like a mitt on your hand so that there are no loose ends.	
——	——	——	15. Lay a towel across patient's chest and on top of bath blanket.	
——	——	——	16. *With no cleanser on the washcloth, wipe one eye from the inner part of the eye, near the nose, to the outer part. Rinse or turn the cloth before washing the other eye.*	
——	——	——	17. Bathe patient's face, neck, and ears. Apply appropriate emollient.	
——	——	——	18. Expose patient's far arm and place towel lengthwise under it. Using firm strokes, wash hand, arm, and axilla, lifting the arm as necessary to access axillary region. Rinse, if necessary, and dry. Apply appropriate emollient.	
——	——	——	19. Place a folded towel on the bed next to the patient's hand and put basin on it. Soak the patient's hand in basin. Wash, rinse if necessary, and dry hand. Apply appropriate emollient.	
——	——	——	20. Repeat Actions 18 and 19 for the arm nearer you. An option for the shorter nurse or one prone to back strain might be to bathe one side of the patient and move to the other side of the bed to complete the bath.	
——	——	——	21. Spread a towel across patient's chest. Lower bath blanket to patient's umbilical area. Wash, rinse, if necessary, and dry chest. Keep chest covered with towel between the wash and rinse. Pay special attention to the folds of skin under the breasts.	
——	——	——	22. Lower bath blanket to the perineal area. Place a towel over patient's chest.	
——	——	——	23. Wash; rinse, if necessary; and dry abdomen. Carefully inspect and clean umbilical area and any abdominal folds or creases.	
——	——	——	24. Return bath blanket to original position and expose far leg. Place towel under far leg. Using firm strokes, wash; rinse, if necessary; and dry leg from ankle to knee and knee to groin. Apply appropriate emollient.	

SKILL 31-1

Giving a Bed Bath *(Continued)*

Excellent	Satisfactory	Needs Practice		Comments
——	——	——	25. Wash, rinse if necessary, and dry the foot. Pay particular attention to the areas between toes. Apply appropriate emollient.	
——	——	——	26. Repeat Actions 24 and 25 for the other leg and foot.	
——	——	——	27. Make sure patient is covered with bath blanket. Change water and washcloth at this point or earlier if necessary.	
——	——	——	28. Assist patient to prone or side-lying position. Put on gloves, if not applied earlier. Position bath blanket and towel to expose only the back and buttocks.	
——	——	——	29. Wash; rinse, if necessary; and dry back and buttocks area. *Pay particular attention to cleansing between gluteal folds, and observe for any redness or skin breakdown in the sacral area.*	
——	——	——	30. If not contraindicated, give patient a backrub, as described in Chapter 10. Back massage may be given also after perineal care. Apply appropriate emollient and/or skin barrier product.	
——	——	——	31. Raise the side rail. Refill basin with clean water. Discard washcloth and towel. Remove gloves and put on clean gloves.	
——	——	——	32. Clean perineal area or set up patient so that he or she can complete perineal self-care. If the patient is unable, lower the side rail and complete perineal care, following guidelines in the chapter text. Apply skin barrier, as indicated. Raise side rail, remove gloves, and perform hand hygiene.	
——	——	——	33. Help patient put on a clean gown and assist with the use of other personal toiletries, such as deodorant or cosmetics.	
——	——	——	34. Protect pillow with towel and groom patient's hair.	
——	——	——	35. *When finished, make sure the patient is comfortable, with the side rails up and the bed in the lowest position.*	
——	——	——	36. Change bed linens, as described in Skills 31-4 and 31-5. Dispose of soiled linens according to agency policy. Remove gloves and any other PPE, if used. Perform hand hygiene.	

Skill Checklists for Fundamentals of Nursing:
The Art and Science of Nursing Care, 7th edition

Name _____   Date _____

Unit _____   Position _____

Instructor/Evaluator: _____   Position _____

SKILL 31-2

Assisting the Patient With Oral Care

Goal: The patient will have a clean mouth and clean teeth, exhibit a positive body image, and verbalize the importance of oral care.

Excellent	Satisfactory	Needs Practice		Comments
——	——	——	1. Perform hand hygiene and put on gloves if assisting with oral care, and/or other PPE, if indicated.	
——	——	——	2. Identify the patient. Explain procedure to patient.	
——	——	——	3. Assemble equipment on overbed table within patient's reach.	
——	——	——	4. Close the room door or curtains. Place the bed at an appropriate and comfortable working height, usually elbow height of the caregiver (VISN 8, 2009).	
——	——	——	5. Lower side rail and assist patient to sitting position if permitted, or turn patient onto side. Place towel across patient's chest. Raise bed to a comfortable working position.	
——	——	——	6. Encourage patient to brush own teeth, or assist if necessary.	
——	——	——	a. Moisten toothbrush and apply toothpaste to bristles.	
——	——	——	b. Place brush at a 45-degree angle to gum line and brush from gum line to crown of each tooth. Brush outer and inner surfaces. Brush back and forth across biting surface of each tooth.	
——	——	——	c. Brush tongue gently with toothbrush.	
——	——	——	d. Have patient rinse vigorously with water and spit into emesis basin. Repeat until clear. Suction may be used as an alternative for removal of fluid and secretions from mouth.	
——	——	——	7. Assist patient to floss teeth, if appropriate:	
——	——	——	a. Remove approximately 6″ of dental floss from container or use a plastic floss holder. Wrap the floss around the index fingers, keeping about 1″ to 1.5″ of floss taut between the fingers.	
——	——	——	b. Insert floss gently between teeth, moving it back and forth downward to the gums.	
——	——	——	c. Move the floss up and down, first on one side of a tooth and then on the side of the other tooth, until the surfaces are clean. Repeat in the spaces between all teeth.	
——	——	——	d. Instruct patient to rinse mouth well with water after flossing.	

SKILL 31-2

Assisting the Patient With Oral Care *(Continued)*

Excellent	Satisfactory	Needs Practice		Comments
___	___	___	8. Offer mouthwash if patient prefers.	
___	___	___	9. Offer lip balm or petroleum jelly.	
___	___	___	10. Remove equipment. Remove gloves and discard. Raise side rail and lower bed. Assist patient to a position of comfort.	
___	___	___	11. Remove any other PPE, if used. Perform hand hygiene.	

Skill Checklists for Fundamentals of Nursing:
The Art and Science of Nursing Care, 7th edition

Name _____ Date _____

Unit _____ Position _____

Instructor/Evaluator: _____ Position _____

SKILL 31-3

Providing Oral Care for the Dependent Patient

Goal: The patient's mouth and teeth will be clean; the patient will not experience impaired oral mucous membranes; the patient will demonstrate improvement in body image; and the patient will verbalize, if able, an understanding about the importance of oral care.

Excellent	Satisfactory	Needs Practice		Comments
——	——	——	1. Perform hand hygiene and put on PPE, if indicated.	
——	——	——	2. Identify the patient. Explain procedure to patient.	
——	——	——	3. Assemble equipment on overbed table within reach.	
——	——	——	4. Close the room door or curtains. Place the bed at an appropriate and comfortable working height, usually elbow height of the caregiver (VISN 8, 2009). Lower one side rail and position patient on the side, with head tilted forward. Place towel across patient's chest and emesis basin in position under chin. Put on gloves.	
——	——	——	5. Gently open the patient's mouth by applying pressure to lower jaw at the front of the mouth. Remove dentures, if present. Brush the teeth and gums carefully with toothbrush and paste. Lightly brush the tongue.	
——	——	——	6. Use toothette dipped in water to rinse the oral cavity. If desired, insert the rubber tip of the irrigating syringe into patient's mouth and rinse gently with a small amount of water. *Position patient's head to allow for return of water or use suction apparatus to remove the water from oral cavity.*	
——	——	——	7. Clean the dentures before replacing.	
——	——	——	8. Apply lubricant to patient's lips.	
——	——	——	9. Remove equipment and return patient to a position of comfort. Remove your gloves. Raise side rail and lower bed.	
——	——	——	10. Remove additional PPE, if used. Perform hand hygiene.	

Skill Checklists for Fundamentals of Nursing:
The Art and Science of Nursing Care, 7th edition

Name _____   Date _____

Unit _____   Position _____

Instructor/Evaluator: _____   Position _____

Excellent	Satisfactory	Needs Practice	SKILL 31-4 **Making an Unoccupied Bed**	Comments
			Goal: The bed linens will be changed without injury to the nurse or patient.	
___	___	___	1. Assemble equipment and arrange on a bedside chair in the order in which items will be used.	
___	___	___	2. Perform hand hygiene. Put on PPE, as indicated.	
___	___	___	3. Adjust the bed to a comfortable working height, usually elbow height of the caregiver (VISN 8, 2009). Drop the side rails.	
___	___	___	4. Disconnect call bell or any tubes from bed linens.	
___	___	___	5. Put on gloves. Loosen all linen as you move around the bed, from the head of the bed on the far side to the head of the bed on the near side.	
___	___	___	6. Fold reusable linens, such as sheets, blankets, or spread, in place on the bed in fourths and hang them over a clean chair.	
___	___	___	7. Snugly roll all the soiled linen inside the bottom sheet and place directly into the laundry hamper. *Do not place on floor or furniture. Do not hold soiled linens against your uniform.*	
___	___	___	8. If possible, shift mattress up to head of bed. If mattress is soiled, clean and dry according to facility policy before applying new sheets.	
___	___	___	9. Remove your gloves, unless indicated for transmission precautions. Place the bottom sheet with its center fold in the center of the bed. Open the sheet and fan-fold to the center.	
___	___	___	10. If using, place the drawsheet with its center fold in the center of the bed and positioned so it will be located under the patient's midsection. Open the drawsheet and fan-fold to the center of the mattress. If a protective pad is used, place it over the drawsheet in the proper area and open to the center fold. Not all agencies use drawsheets routinely. The nurse may decide to use one. In some institutions, the protective pad doubles as a drawsheet.	
___	___	___	11. Pull the bottom sheet over the corners at the head and foot of the mattress. Tuck the drawsheet securely under the mattress.	

SKILL 31-4
Making an Unoccupied Bed *(Continued)*

Excellent	Satisfactory	Needs Practice		Comments
——	——	——	12. Move to the other side of the bed to secure bottom linens. Pull the bottom sheet tightly and secure over the corners at the head and foot of the mattress. Pull the drawsheet tightly and tuck it securely under the mattress.	
——	——	——	13. Place the top sheet on the bed with its center fold in the center of the bed and with the hem even with the head of the mattress. Unfold the top sheet. Follow same procedure with top blanket or spread, placing the upper edge about 6″ below the top of the sheet.	
——	——	——	14. Tuck the top sheet and blanket under the foot of the bed on the near side. Miter the corners.	
——	——	——	15. Fold the upper 6″ of the top sheet down over the spread and make a cuff.	
——	——	——	16. Move to the other side of the bed and follow the same procedure for securing top sheets under the foot of the bed and making a cuff.	
——	——	——	17. Place the pillows on the bed. Open each pillowcase in the same manner as you opened other linens. Gather the pillowcase over one hand toward the closed end. Grasp the pillow with the hand inside the pillowcase. Keep a firm hold on the top of the pillow and pull the cover onto the pillow. Place the pillow at the head of the bed.	
——	——	——	18. Fan-fold or pie-fold the top linens.	
——	——	——	19. Secure the signal device on the bed according to agency policy.	
——	——	——	20. Raise side rail and lower bed.	
——	——	——	21. Dispose of soiled linen according to agency policy.	
——	——	——	22. Remove any other PPE, if used. Perform hand hygiene.	

58

Skill Checklists for Fundamentals of Nursing:
The Art and Science of Nursing Care, 7th edition

Name _____ Date _____

Unit _____ Position _____

Instructor/Evaluator: _____ Position _____

Excellent	Satisfactory	Needs Practice	SKILL 31-5 **Making an Occupied Bed** **Goal:** The bed linens are applied without injury to the patient or nurse.	Comments
____	____	____	1. Check chart for limitations on patient's physical activity.	
____	____	____	2. Assemble equipment and arrange on bedside chair in the order the items will be used.	
____	____	____	3. Perform hand hygiene. Put on PPE, as indicated.	
____	____	____	4. Identify the patient. Explain what you are going to do.	
____	____	____	5. Close curtains around bed and close door to room if possible.	
____	____	____	6. Adjust the bed to a comfortable working height, usually elbow height of the caregiver (VISN 8, 2006).	
____	____	____	7. Lower side rail nearest you, leaving the opposite side rail up. Place bed in flat position unless contraindicated.	
____	____	____	8. Put on gloves. Check bed linens for patient's personal items. ***Disconnect the call bell or any tubes/drains from bed linens.***	
____	____	____	9. Place a bath blanket over patient. Have patient hold on to bath blanket while you reach under it and remove top linens. Leave top sheet in place if a bath blanket is not used. Fold linen that is to be reused over the back of a chair. Discard soiled linen in laundry bag or hamper. ***Do not place on floor or furniture. Do not hold soiled linens against your uniform.***	
____	____	____	10. If possible and another person is available to assist, grasp mattress securely and shift it up to head of bed.	
____	____	____	11. Assist patient to turn toward opposite side of the bed, and reposition pillow under patient's head.	
____	____	____	12. Loosen all bottom linens from head, foot, and side of bed.	
____	____	____	13. Fan-fold soiled linens as close to patient as possible.	
____	____	____	14. Use clean linen and make the near side of the bed. Place the bottom sheet with its center fold in the center of the bed. Open the sheet and fan-fold to the center, positioning it under the old linens. Pull the bottom sheet over the corners at the head and foot of the mattress.	

Copyright © 2011 by Wolters Kluwer Health | Lippincott Williams & Wilkins. *Skill Checklists for Fundamentals of Nursing: The Art and Science of Nursing Care*, 7th edition, by Carol Taylor, Carol Lillis, Priscilla LeMone, Pamela Lynn, and Marilee LeBon.

Making an Occupied Bed *(Continued)*

Excellent	Satisfactory	Needs Practice		Comments
——	——	——	15. If using, place the drawsheet with its center fold in the center of the bed and positioned so it will be located under the patient's midsection. Open the drawsheet and fan-fold to the center of the mattress. Tuck the drawsheet securely under the mattress. If a protective pad is used, place it over the drawsheet in the proper area and open to the center fold. Not all agencies use drawsheets routinely. The nurse may decide to use one.	
——	——	——	16. Raise side rail. Assist patient to roll over the folded linen in the middle of the bed toward you. Reposition pillow and bath blanket or top sheet. Move to other side of the bed and lower side rail.	
——	——	——	17. Loosen and remove all bottom linen. Discard soiled linen in laundry bag or hamper. *Do not place on floor or furniture. Do not hold soiled linens against your uniform.*	
——	——	——	18. Ease clean linen from under the patient. Pull the bottom sheet taut and secure at the corners at the head and foot of the mattress. Pull the drawsheet tight and smooth. Tuck the drawsheet securely under the mattress.	
——	——	——	19. Assist patient to turn back to the center of bed. Remove pillow and change pillowcase. Open each pillowcase in the same manner as you opened other linens. Gather the pillowcase over one hand toward the closed end. Grasp the pillow with the hand inside the pillowcase. Keep a firm hold on the top of the pillow and pull the cover onto the pillow. Place the pillow under the patient's head.	
——	——	——	20. Apply top linen, sheet, and blanket if desired, so that it is centered. Fold the top linens over at the patient's shoulders to make a cuff. Have patient hold on to top linen and remove the bath blanket from underneath.	
——	——	——	21. Secure top linens under foot of mattress and miter corners. Loosen top linens over patient's feet by grasping them in the area of the feet and pulling gently toward foot of bed.	
——	——	——	22. Return patient to a position of comfort. Remove your gloves. Raise side rail and lower bed. Reattach call bell.	
——	——	——	23. Dispose of soiled linens according to agency policy.	
——	——	——	24. Remove any other PPE, if used. Perform hand hygiene.	

Skill Checklists for Fundamentals of Nursing:
The Art and Science of Nursing Care, 7th edition

Name _____ Date _____

Unit _____ Position _____

Instructor/Evaluator: _____ Position _____

Skill 32-1

Cleaning a Wound and Applying a Dry, Sterile Dressing

Excellent	Satisfactory	Needs Practice	**Goal:** The wound is cleaned and protected with a dressing without contaminating the wound area, without causing trauma to the wound, and without causing the patient to experience pain or discomfort.	Comments
___	___	___	1. Review the medical orders for wound care or the nursing plan of care related to wound care.	
___	___	___	2. Gather the necessary supplies and bring to the bedside stand or overbed table.	
___	___	___	3. Perform hand hygiene and put on PPE, if indicated.	
___	___	___	4. Identify the patient.	
___	___	___	5. Close curtains around bed and close door to room if possible. Explain what you are going to do and why you are going to do it to the patient.	
___	___	___	6. Assess the patient for possible need for nonpharmacologic pain-reducing interventions or analgesic medication before wound care dressing change. Administer appropriate prescribed analgesic. Allow enough time for analgesic to achieve its effectiveness.	
___	___	___	7. Place a waste receptacle or bag at a convenient location for use during the procedure.	
___	___	___	8. Adjust bed to comfortable working height, usually elbow height of the caregiver (VISN 8, 2009).	
___	___	___	9. Assist the patient to a comfortable position that provides easy access to the wound area. Use the bath blanket to cover any exposed area other than the wound. Place a waterproof pad under the wound site.	
___	___	___	10. Check the position of drains, tubes, or other adjuncts before removing the dressing. Put on clean, disposable gloves and loosen tape on the old dressings. If necessary, use an adhesive remover to help get the tape off.	
___	___	___	11. Carefully remove the soiled dressings. If there is resistance, use a silicone-based adhesive remover to help remove the tape. If any part of the dressing sticks to the underlying skin, use small amounts of sterile saline to help loosen and remove.	

Excellent	Satisfactory	Needs Practice	Skill 32-1 **Cleaning a Wound and Applying a Dry, Sterile Dressing** *(Continued)*
			Comments
——	——	——	12. After removing the dressing, note the presence, amount, type, color, and odor of any drainage on the dressings. Place soiled dressings in the appropriate waste receptacle. Remove your gloves and dispose of them in an appropriate waste receptacle.
——	——	——	13. Inspect the wound site for size, appearance, and drainage. Assess if any pain is present. Check the status of sutures, adhesive closure strips, staples, and drains or tubes, if present. Note any problems to include in your documentation.
——	——	——	14. *Using sterile technique, prepare a sterile work area and open the needed supplies.*
——	——	——	15. Open the sterile cleaning solution. Depending on the amount of cleaning needed, the solution might be poured directly over gauze sponges over a container for small cleaning jobs, or into a basin for more complex or larger cleaning.
——	——	——	16. Put on sterile gloves.
——	——	——	17. Clean the wound. *Clean the wound from top to bottom and from the center to the outside. Following this pattern, use new gauze for each wipe, placing the used gauze in the waste receptacle. Alternately, spray the wound from top to bottom with a commercially prepared wound cleanser.*
——	——	——	18. Once the wound is cleaned, dry the area using a gauze sponge in the same manner. Apply ointment or perform other treatments, as ordered.
——	——	——	19. If a drain is in use at the wound location, clean around the drain.
——	——	——	20. Apply a layer of dry, sterile dressing over the wound. Forceps may be used to apply the dressing.
——	——	——	21. Place a second layer of gauze over the wound site.
——	——	——	22. Apply a surgical or abdominal pad (ABD) over the gauze at the site as the outermost layer of the dressing.
——	——	——	23. Remove and discard gloves. Apply tape, Montgomery straps, or roller gauze to secure the dressings. Alternately, many commercial wound products are self-adhesive and do not require additional tape.
——	——	——	24. After securing the dressing, label dressing with date and time. Remove all remaining equipment; place the patient in a comfortable position, with side rails up and bed in the lowest position.

Skill 32-1

Cleaning a Wound and Applying a Dry, Sterile Dressing *(Continued)*

Excellent	Satisfactory	Needs Practice		Comments
——	——	——	25. Remove PPE, if used. Perform hand hygiene.	
——	——	——	26. Check all wound dressings every shift. More frequent checks may be needed if the wound is more complex or dressings become saturated quickly.	

Skill Checklists for Fundamentals of Nursing:
The Art and Science of Nursing Care, 7th edition

Name _____ Date _____

Unit _____ Position _____

Instructor/Evaluator: _____ Position _____

Excellent	Satisfactory	Needs Practice	SKILL 32-2 **Applying a Saline-Moistened Dressing**	Comments
			Goal: The procedure is accomplished without contaminating the wound area, without causing trauma to the wound, and without causing the patient to experience pain or discomfort.	
——	——	——	1. Review the medical orders for wound care or the nursing plan of care related to wound care.	
——	——	——	2. Gather the necessary supplies and bring to the bedside stand or overbed table.	
——	——	——	3. Perform hand hygiene and put on PPE, if indicated.	
——	——	——	4. Identify the patient.	
——	——	——	5. Close curtains around bed and close door to room if possible. Explain what you are going to do and why you are going to do it to the patient.	
——	——	——	6. Assess the patient for possible need for nonpharmacologic pain-reducing interventions or analgesic medication before wound care dressing change. Administer appropriate prescribed analgesic. Allow enough time for analgesic to achieve its effectiveness.	
——	——	——	7. Place a waste receptacle or bag at a convenient location for use during the procedure.	
——	——	——	8. Adjust bed to comfortable working height, usually elbow height of the caregiver (VISN 8, 2009).	
——	——	——	9. Assist the patient to a comfortable position that provides easy access to the wound area. Position the patient so the wound cleanser or irrigation solution will flow from the clean end of the wound toward the dirtier end, if being used (see Skill 32-3 for irrigation techniques). Use the bath blanket to cover any exposed area other than the wound. Place a waterproof pad under the wound site.	
——	——	——	10. Put on clean gloves. Carefully and gently remove the soiled dressings. If there is resistance, use a silicone-based adhesive remover to help remove the tape. If any part of the dressing sticks to the underlying skin, use small amounts of sterile saline to help loosen and remove.	
——	——	——	11. After removing the dressing, note the presence, amount, type, color, and odor of any drainage on the dressings. Place soiled dressings in the appropriate waste receptacle.	

Excellent	Satisfactory	Needs Practice		Comments

SKILL 32-2
Applying a Saline-Moistened Dressing *(Continued)*

Excellent	Satisfactory	Needs Practice		
___	___	___	12. Assess the wound for appearance, stage, the presence of eschar, granulation tissue, epithelialization, undermining, tunneling, necrosis, sinus tract, and drainage. Assess the appearance of the surrounding tissue. Measure the wound.	
___	___	___	13. Remove your gloves and put them in the receptacle.	
___	___	___	14. Using sterile technique, open the supplies and dressings. Place the fine-mesh gauze into the basin and pour the ordered solution over the mesh to saturate it.	
___	___	___	15. Put on the sterile gloves. Alternately, clean gloves (clean technique) may be used to clean a chronic wound.	
___	___	___	16. Clean the wound. Refer to Skill 32-1. Alternately, irrigate the wound, as ordered or required (see Skill 32-3).	
___	___	___	17. Dry the surrounding skin with sterile gauze dressings.	
___	___	___	18. Apply a skin protectant to the surrounding skin, if needed.	
___	___	___	19. If not already on, put on sterile gloves. Squeeze excess fluid from the gauze dressing. Unfold and fluff the dressing.	
___	___	___	20. Gently press to loosely pack the moistened gauze into the wound. If necessary, use the forceps or cotton-tipped applicators to press the gauze into all wound surfaces.	
___	___	___	21. Apply several dry, sterile gauze pads over the wet gauze.	
___	___	___	22. Place the ABD pad over the gauze.	
___	___	___	23. Remove and discard gloves. Apply tape, Montgomery straps, or roller gauze to secure the dressings. Alternately, many commercial wound products are self-adhesive and do not require additional tape.	
___	___	___	24. After securing the dressing, label dressing with date and time. Remove all remaining equipment; place the patient in a comfortable position, with side rails up and bed in the lowest position.	
___	___	___	25. Remove PPE, if used. Perform hand hygiene.	
___	___	___	26. Check all wound dressings every shift. More frequent checks may be needed if the wound is more complex or dressings become saturated quickly.	

Skill Checklists for Fundamentals of Nursing:
The Art and Science of Nursing Care, 7th edition

Name _____   Date _____

Unit _____   Position _____

Instructor/Evaluator: _____   Position _____

Excellent	Satisfactory	Needs Practice	SKILL 32-3 **Performing Irrigation of a Wound**	Comments
			Goal: The wound is cleaned without contamination or trauma and without causing the patient to experience pain or discomfort.	
——	——	——	1. Review the medical orders for wound care or the nursing plan of care related to wound care.	
——	——	——	2. Gather the necessary supplies and bring to the bedside stand or overbed table.	
——	——	——	3. Perform hand hygiene and put on PPE, if indicated.	
——	——	——	4. Identify the patient.	
——	——	——	5. Close curtains around bed and close door to room if possible. Explain what you are going to do and why you are going to do it to the patient.	
——	——	——	6. Assess the patient for possible need for nonpharmacologic pain-reducing interventions or analgesic medication before wound care and/or dressing change. Administer appropriate prescribed analgesic. Allow enough time for analgesic to achieve its effectiveness before beginning procedure.	
——	——	——	7. Place a waste receptacle or bag at a convenient location for use during the procedure.	
——	——	——	8. Adjust bed to comfortable working height, usually elbow height of the caregiver (VISN 8, 2009).	
——	——	——	9. Assist the patient to a comfortable position that provides easy access to the wound area. Position the patient so the irrigation solution will flow from the clean end of the wound toward the dirtier end. Use the bath blanket to cover any exposed area other than the wound. Place a waterproof pad under the wound site.	
——	——	——	10. Put on a gown, mask, and eye protection.	
——	——	——	11. Put on clean gloves. Carefully and gently remove the soiled dressings. If there is resistance, use a silicone-based adhesive remover to help remove the tape. If any part of the dressing sticks to the underlying skin, use small amounts of sterile saline to help loosen and remove.	
——	——	——	12. After removing the dressing, note the presence, amount, type, color, and odor of any drainage on the dressings. Place soiled dressings in the appropriate waste receptacle.	

SKILL 32-3
Performing Irrigation of a Wound *(Continued)*

Excellent	Satisfactory	Needs Practice		Comments
— — —			13. Assess the wound for appearance, stage, the presence of eschar, granulation tissue, epithelialization, undermining, tunneling, necrosis, sinus tract, and drainage. Assess the appearance of the surrounding tissue. Measure the wound.	
— — —			14. Remove your gloves and put them in the receptacle.	
— — —			15. Set up a sterile field, if indicated, and wound cleaning supplies. Pour warmed sterile irrigating solution into the sterile container. Put on the sterile gloves. Alternately, clean gloves (clean technique) may be used when irrigating a chronic wound.	
— — —			16. Position the sterile basin below the wound to collect the irrigation fluid.	
— — —			17. Fill the irrigation syringe with solution. *Using your nondominant hand, gently apply pressure to the basin against the skin below the wound to form a seal with the skin.*	
— — —			18. *Gently direct a stream of solution into the wound. Keep the tip of the syringe at least 1 inch above the upper tip of the wound. When using a catheter tip, insert it gently into the wound until it meets resistance. Gently flush all wound areas.*	
— — —			19. Watch for the solution to flow smoothly and evenly. When the solution from the wound flows out clear, discontinue irrigation.	
— — —			20. Dry the surrounding skin with gauze dressings.	
— — —			21. Apply a skin protectant to the surrounding skin.	
— — —			22. Apply a new dressing to the wound (see Skill 32-1).	
— — —			23. Remove and discard gloves. Apply tape, Montgomery straps, or roller gauze to secure the dressings. Alternately, many commercial wound products are self-adhesive and do not require additional tape.	
— — —			24. After securing the dressing, label dressing with date and time. Remove all remaining equipment; place the patient in a comfortable position, with side rails up and bed in the lowest position.	
— — —			25. Remove remaining PPE. Perform hand hygiene.	
— — —			26. Check all wound dressings every shift. More frequent checks may be needed if the wound is more complex or dressings become saturated quickly.	

Skill Checklists for Fundamentals of Nursing:
The Art and Science of Nursing Care, 7th edition

Name _____ Date _____

Unit _____ Position _____

Instructor/Evaluator: _____ Position _____

Excellent	Satisfactory	Needs Practice	SKILL 32-4 **Caring for a Jackson-Pratt Drain**	
			Goal: The drain is patent and intact.	**Comments**
—	—	—	1. Review the medical orders for wound care or the nursing plan of care related to wound/drain care.	
—	—	—	2. Gather the necessary supplies and bring to the bedside stand or overbed table.	
—	—	—	3. Perform hand hygiene and put on PPE, if indicated.	
—	—	—	4. Identify the patient.	
—	—	—	5. Close curtains around bed and close door to room if possible. Explain what you are going to do and why you are going to do it to the patient.	
—	—	—	6. Assess the patient for possible need for nonpharmacologic pain-reducing interventions or analgesic medication before wound care dressing change. Administer appropriate prescribed analgesic. Allow enough time for analgesic to achieve its effectiveness before beginning procedure.	
—	—	—	7. Place a waste receptacle at a convenient location for use during the procedure.	
—	—	—	8. Adjust bed to comfortable working height, usually elbow height of the caregiver (VISN 8, 2009).	
—	—	—	9. Assist the patient to a comfortable position that provides easy access to the drain and/or wound area. Use a bath blanket to cover any exposed area other than the wound. Place a waterproof pad under the wound site.	
—	—	—	10. Put on clean gloves; put on mask or face shield if indicated.	
—	—	—	11. Place the graduated collection container under the outlet of the drain. Without contaminating the outlet valve, pull the cap off. The chamber will expand completely as it draws in air. *Empty the chamber's contents completely into the container. Use the gauze pad to clean the outlet. Fully compress the chamber with one hand and replace the cap with your other hand.*	
—	—	—	12. Check the patency of the equipment. Make sure the tubing is free from twists and kinks.	
—	—	—	13. Secure the Jackson-Pratt drain to the patient's gown below the wound with a safety pin, making sure that there is no tension on the tubing.	

Excellent	Satisfactory	Needs Practice	

SKILL 32-4

Caring for a Jackson-Pratt Drain *(Continued)*

Comments

Excellent	Satisfactory	Needs Practice		Comments
___	___	___	14. Carefully measure and record the character, color, and amount of the drainage. Discard the drainage according to facility policy. Remove gloves.	
___	___	___	15. Put on clean gloves. If the drain site has a dressing, redress the site. Include cleaning of the sutures with the gauze pad moistened with normal saline. Dry sutures with gauze before applying new dressing.	
___	___	___	16. If the drain site is open to air, observe the sutures that secure the drain to the skin. Look for signs of pulling, tearing, swelling, or infection of the surrounding skin. Gently clean the sutures with the gauze pad moistened with normal saline. Dry with a new gauze pad. Apply skin protectant to the surrounding skin if needed.	
___	___	___	17. Remove and discard gloves. Remove all remaining equipment; place the patient in a comfortable position, with side rails up and bed in the lowest position.	
___	___	___	18. Remove additional PPE, if used. Perform hand hygiene.	
___	___	___	19. Check drain status at least every 4 hours. Check all wound dressings every shift. More frequent checks may be needed if the wound is more complex or dressings become saturated quickly.	

Skill Checklists for Fundamentals of Nursing:
The Art and Science of Nursing Care, 7th edition

Name _____ Date _____

Unit _____ Position _____

Instructor/Evaluator: _____ Position _____

Excellent	Satisfactory	Needs Practice	SKILL 32-5 **Caring for a Hemovac Drain**	
			Goal: The drain is patent and intact.	**Comments**
——	——	——	1. Review the medical orders for wound care or the nursing plan of care related to wound/drain care.	
——	——	——	2. Gather the necessary supplies and bring to the bedside stand or overbed table.	
——	——	——	3. Perform hand hygiene and put on PPE, if indicated.	
——	——	——	4. Identify the patient.	
——	——	——	5. Close curtains around bed and close door to room if possible. Explain what you are going to do and why you are going to do it to the patient.	
——	——	——	6. Assess the patient for possible need for nonpharmacologic pain-reducing interventions or analgesic medication before wound care dressing change. Administer appropriate prescribed analgesic. Allow enough time for analgesic to achieve its effectiveness before beginning procedure.	
——	——	——	7. Place a waste receptacle at a convenient location for use during the procedure.	
——	——	——	8. Adjust bed to comfortable working height, usually elbow height of the caregiver (VISN 8, 2009).	
——	——	——	9. Assist the patient to a comfortable position that provides easy access to the drain and/or wound area. Use a bath blanket to cover any exposed area other than the wound. Place a waterproof pad under the wound site.	
——	——	——	10. Put on clean gloves; put on mask or face shield if indicated.	
——	——	——	11. Place the graduated collection container under the outlet of the drain. Without contaminating the outlet, pull the cap off. The chamber will expand completely as it draws in air. *Empty the chamber's contents completely into the container. Use the gauze pad to clean the outlet. Fully compress the chamber by pushing the top and bottom together with your hands. Keep the device tightly compressed while you apply the cap.*	
——	——	——	12. Check the patency of the equipment. Make sure the tubing is free from twists and kinks.	

SKILL 32-5

Caring for a Hemovac Drain *(Continued)*

Excellent	Satisfactory	Needs Practice		Comments
——	——	——	13. Secure the Hemovac drain to the patient's gown below the wound with a safety pin, making sure that there is no tension on the tubing.	
——	——	——	14. Carefully measure and record the character, color, and amount of the drainage. Discard the drainage according to facility policy.	
——	——	——	15. Put on clean gloves. If the drain site has a dressing, redress the site. Include cleaning of the sutures with the gauze pad moistened with normal saline. Dry sutures with gauze before applying new dressing.	
——	——	——	16. If the drain site is open to air, observe the sutures that secure the drain to the skin. Look for signs of pulling, tearing, swelling, or infection of the surrounding skin. Gently clean the sutures with the gauze pad moistened with normal saline. Dry with a new gauze pad. Apply skin protectant to the surrounding skin if needed.	
——	——	——	17. Remove and discard gloves. Remove all remaining equipment; place the patient in a comfortable position, with side rails up and bed in the lowest position.	
——	——	——	18. Remove additional PPE, if used. Perform hand hygiene.	
——	——	——	19. Check drain status at least every 4 hours. Check all wound dressings every shift. More frequent checks may be needed if the wound is more complex or dressings become saturated quickly.	

Skill Checklists for Fundamentals of Nursing:
The Art and Science of Nursing Care, 7th edition

Name _____   Date _____

Unit _____   Position _____

Instructor/Evaluator: _____   Position _____

Excellent	Satisfactory	Needs Practice	SKILL 32-6 **Collecting a Wound Culture**	Comments
			Goal: The culture is obtained without evidence of contamination, without exposing the patient to additional pathogens, and without causing discomfort for the patient.	
___	___	___	1. Review the medical orders for obtaining a wound culture.	
___	___	___	2. Gather the necessary supplies and bring to the bedside stand or overbed table.	
___	___	___	3. Perform hand hygiene and put on PPE, if indicated.	
___	___	___	4. Identify the patient.	
___	___	___	5. Close curtains around bed and close door to room if possible. Explain what you are going to do and why you are going to do it to the patient.	
___	___	___	6. Assess the patient for possible need for nonpharmacologic pain-reducing interventions or analgesic medication before obtaining the wound culture. Administer appropriate prescribed analgesic. Allow enough time for analgesic to achieve its effectiveness before beginning procedure.	
___	___	___	7. Place an appropriate waste receptacle within easy reach for use during the procedure.	
___	___	___	8. Adjust bed to comfortable working height, usually elbow height of the caregiver (VISN 8, 2009).	
___	___	___	9. Assist the patient to a comfortable position that provides easy access to the wound. If necessary, drape the patient with the bath blanket to expose only the wound area. Place a waterproof pad under the wound site. Check the culture label against the patient's identification bracelet.	
___	___	___	10. If there is a dressing in place on the wound, put on clean gloves. Carefully and gently remove the soiled dressings. If there is resistance, use a silicone-based adhesive remover to help remove the tape. If any part of the dressing sticks to the underlying skin, use small amounts of sterile saline to help loosen and remove.	
___	___	___	11. After removing the dressing, note the presence, amount, type, color, and odor of any drainage on the dressings. Place soiled dressings in the appropriate waste receptacle.	
___	___	___	12. Assess the wound for appearance, stage, the presence of eschar, granulation tissue, epithelialization, undermining, tunneling, necrosis, sinus tract, and drainage. Assess the appearance of the surrounding tissue. Measure the wound.	

Excellent	Satisfactory	Needs Practice	SKILL 32-6 **Collecting a Wound Culture** *(Continued)*	
				Comments
——	——	——	13. Remove your gloves and put them in the receptacle.	
——	——	——	14. Set up a sterile field, if indicated, and wound cleaning supplies. Put on the sterile gloves. Alternately, clean gloves (clean technique) may be used when cleaning a chronic wound.	
——	——	——	15. Clean the wound. Refer to Skill 32-1. Alternately, irrigate the wound, as ordered or required (see Skill 32-3).	
——	——	——	16. Dry the surrounding skin with gauze dressings. Put on clean gloves.	
——	——	——	17. Twist the cap to loosen the swab on the Culturette tube, or open the separate swab and remove the cap from the culture tube. *Keep the swab and inside of the culture tube sterile.*	
——	——	——	18. If contact with the wound is necessary to separate wound margins to permit insertion of the swab deep into the wound, put a sterile glove on one hand to manipulate the wound margins. Clean gloves may be appropriate for contact with pressure ulcers and chronic wounds.	
——	——	——	19. *Carefully insert the swab into the wound. Press and rotate the swab several times over the wound surfaces. Avoid touching the swab to intact skin at the wound edges. Use another swab if collecting a specimen from another site.*	
——	——	——	20. Place the swab back in the culture tube. *Do not touch the outside of the tube with the swab.* Secure the cap. Some swab containers have an ampule of medium at the bottom of the tube. It might be necessary to crush this ampule to activate. Follow the manufacturer's instructions for use.	
——	——	——	21. Remove gloves and discard them accordingly.	
——	——	——	22. Put on gloves. Place a dressing on the wound, as appropriate, based on medical orders and/or the nursing plan of care. Remove gloves.	
——	——	——	23. After securing the dressing, label dressing with date and time. Remove all remaining equipment; place the patient in a comfortable position, with side rails up and bed in the lowest position.	
——	——	——	24. Label the specimen according to your institution's guidelines and send it to the laboratory in a biohazard bag.	
——	——	——	25. Remove PPE, if used. Perform hand hygiene.	

Skill Checklists for Fundamentals of Nursing:
The Art and Science of Nursing Care, 7th edition

Name _____ Date _____

Unit _____ Position _____

Instructor/Evaluator: _____ Position _____

SKILL 32-7

Applying Negative-Pressure Wound Therapy

Goal: The therapy is accomplished without contaminating the wound area, without causing trauma to the wound, and without causing the patient to experience pain or discomfort.

Excellent	Satisfactory	Needs Practice		Comments
——	——	——	1. Review the medical order for the application of NPWT therapy, including the ordered pressure setting for the device.	
——	——	——	2. Gather the necessary supplies and bring to the bedside stand or overbed table.	
——	——	——	3. Perform hand hygiene and put on PPE, if indicated.	
——	——	——	4. Identify the patient.	
——	——	——	5. Close curtains around bed and close door to room if possible. Explain what you are going to do and why you are going to do it to the patient.	
——	——	——	6. Assess the patient for possible need for nonpharmacologic pain-reducing interventions or analgesic medication before wound care dressing change. Administer appropriate prescribed analgesic. Allow enough time for analgesic to achieve its effectiveness before beginning procedure.	
——	——	——	7. Adjust bed to comfortable working height, usually elbow height of the caregiver (VISN 8, 2009).	
——	——	——	8. Assist the patient to a comfortable position that provides easy access to the wound area. Position the patient so the irrigation solution will flow from the clean end of the wound toward the dirty end. Expose the area and drape the patient with a bath blanket if needed. Put a waterproof pad under the wound area.	
——	——	——	9. Have the disposal bag or waste receptacle within easy reach for use during the procedure.	
——	——	——	10. Using sterile technique, prepare a sterile field and add all the sterile supplies needed for the procedure to the field. Pour warmed, sterile irrigating solution into the sterile container.	
——	——	——	11. Put on a gown, mask, and eye protection.	
——	——	——	12. Put on clean gloves. Carefully and gently remove the dressing. If there is resistance, use a silicone-based adhesive remover to help remove the drape. *Note the number of pieces of foam removed from the wound. Compare with the documented number from the previous dressing change.*	

SKILL 32-7
Applying Negative-Pressure Wound Therapy (Continued)

Excellent	Satisfactory	Needs Practice		Comments
——	——	——	13. Discard the dressings in the receptacle. Remove your gloves and put them in the receptacle.	
——	——	——	14. Put on sterile gloves. Using sterile technique, irrigate the wound (see Skill 32-3).	
——	——	——	15. Clean the area around the skin with normal saline. Dry the surrounding skin with a sterile gauze sponge.	
——	——	——	16. Assess the wound for appearance, stage, the presence of eschar, granulation tissue, epithelialization, undermining, tunneling, necrosis, sinus tract, and drainage. Assess the appearance of the surrounding tissue. Measure the wound.	
——	——	——	17. **Wipe intact skin around the wound with a skin-protectant wipe and allow it to dry well.**	
——	——	——	18. Remove gloves if they become contaminated and discard them into the receptacle.	
——	——	——	19. Put on a new pair of sterile gloves, if necessary. **Using sterile scissors, cut the foam to the shape and measurement of the wound. Do not cut foam over the wound.** More than one piece of foam may be necessary if the first piece is cut too small. Carefully place the foam in the wound. **Ensure foam-to-foam contact if more than one piece is required. Note the number of pieces of foam placed in the wound.**	
——	——	——	20. Trim and place the V.A.C. Drape to cover the foam dressing and an additional 3 to 5 cm border of intact periwound tissue. V.A.C. Drape may be cut into multiple pieces for easier handling.	
——	——	——	21. Choose an appropriate site to apply the T.R.A.C. Pad.	
——	——	——	22. Pinch the Drape and cut a 2 cm hole through the Drape. Apply the T.R.A.C. Pad. Remove V.A.C. Canister from package and insert into the V.A.C. Therapy Unit until it locks into place. Connect T.R.A.C. Pad tubing to canister tubing and check that the clamps on each tube are open. Turn on the power to the V.A.C. Therapy Unit and select the prescribed therapy setting.	
——	——	——	23. Assess the dressing to ensure seal integrity. The dressing should be collapsed, shrinking to the foam and skin.	
——	——	——	24. Remove and discard gloves. Apply tape, Montgomery straps, or roller gauze to secure the dressings. Alternately, many commercial wound products are self-adhesive and do not require additional tape.	
——	——	——	25. Label dressing with date and time. Remove all remaining equipment; place the patient in a comfortable position, with side rails up and bed in the lowest position.	

SKILL 32-7

Applying Negative-Pressure Wound Therapy *(Continued)*

Excellent	Satisfactory	Needs Practice		Comments
——	——	——	26. Remove PPE, if used. Perform hand hygiene.	
——	——	——	27. Check all wound dressings every shift. More frequent checks may be needed if the wound is more complex or dressings become saturated quickly.	

Skill Checklists for Fundamentals of Nursing:
The Art and Science of Nursing Care, 7th edition

Name _____   Date _____

Unit _____   Position _____

Instructor/Evaluator: _____   Position _____

SKILL 32-8
Applying an External Heating Pad

Goal: Desired outcome depends on the patient's nursing diagnosis.

Excellent	Satisfactory	Needs Practice		Comments
___	___	___	1. Review the medical order for the application of heat therapy, including frequency, type of therapy, body area to be treated, and length of time for the application.	
___	___	___	2. Gather the necessary supplies and bring to the bedside stand or overbed table.	
___	___	___	3. Perform hand hygiene and put on PPE, if indicated.	
___	___	___	4. Identify the patient.	
___	___	___	5. Close curtains around bed and close door to room if possible. Explain what you are going to do and why you are going to do it to the patient.	
___	___	___	6. Adjust bed to comfortable working height, usually elbow height of the caregiver (VISN 8, 2009).	
___	___	___	7. Assist the patient to a comfortable position that provides easy access to the area where the heat will be applied; use a bath blanket to cover any other exposed area.	
___	___	___	8. Assess the condition of the skin where the heat is to be applied.	
___	___	___	9. Check that the water in the electronic unit is at the appropriate level. Fill the unit two-thirds full or to the fill mark, with distilled water, if necessary. Check the temperature setting on the unit to ensure it is within the safe range.	
___	___	___	10. Attach pad tubing to electronic unit tubing.	
___	___	___	11. Plug in the unit and warm the pad before use. Apply the heating pad to the prescribed area. Secure with gauze bandage or tape.	
___	___	___	12. *Assess the condition of the skin and the patient's response to the heat at frequent intervals, according to facility policy. Do not exceed the prescribed length of time for the application of heat.*	
___	___	___	13. Remove gloves and discard. Remove all remaining equipment; place the patient in a comfortable position, with side rails up and bed in the lowest position.	
___	___	___	14. Remove additional PPE, if used. Perform hand hygiene.	
___	___	___	15. Remove after the prescribed amount of time. Reassess the patient and area of application, noting the effect and presence of adverse effects.	

Skill Checklists for Fundamentals of Nursing:
The Art and Science of Nursing Care, 7th edition

Name _____   Date _____

Unit _____   Position _____

Instructor/Evaluator: _____   Position _____

Excellent	Satisfactory	Needs Practice	SKILL 32-9 **Applying a Warm Compress**	Comments
			Goal: The patient displays signs of improvement, such as decreased inflammation, decreased muscle spasms, or decreased pain that indicate problems have been relieved.	
____	____	____	1. Review the medical order for the application of a moist warm compress, including frequency, and length of time for the application.	
____	____	____	2. Gather the necessary supplies and bring to the bedside stand or overbed table.	
____	____	____	3. Perform hand hygiene and put on PPE, if indicated.	
____	____	____	4. Identify the patient.	
____	____	____	5. Assess the patient for possible need for nonpharmacologic pain-reducing interventions or analgesic medication before beginning the procedure. Administer appropriate analgesic, consulting physician's orders, and allow enough time for analgesic to achieve its effectiveness before beginning procedure.	
____	____	____	6. Close curtains around bed and close door to room if possible. Explain what you are going to do and why you are going to do it to the patient.	
____	____	____	7. If using an electronic heating device, check that the water in the unit is at the appropriate level. Fill the unit two-thirds full with distilled water, or to the fill mark, if necessary. Check the temperature setting on the unit to ensure it is within the safe range. (Refer to Skill 32-8.)	
____	____	____	8. Assist the patient to a comfortable position that provides easy access to the area. Use a bath blanket to cover any exposed area other than the intended site. Place a waterproof pad under the site.	
____	____	____	9. Place a waste receptacle at a convenient location for use during the procedure.	
____	____	____	10. Pour the warmed solution into the container and drop the gauze for the compress into the solution. Alternately, if commercially packaged prewarmed gauze is used, open packaging.	
____	____	____	11. Put on clean gloves. Assess the application site for inflammation, skin color, and ecchymosis.	

SKILL 32-9

Applying a Warm Compress *(Continued)*

Excellent	Satisfactory	Needs Practice		Comments
____	____	____	12. *Retrieve the compress from the warmed solution, squeezing out any excess moisture. Alternately, remove pre-warmed gauze from open package. Apply the compress by gently and carefully molding it to the intended area. Ask patient if the application feels too hot.*	
____	____	____	13. Cover the site with a single layer of gauze and with a clean dry bath towel; secure in place if necessary.	
____	____	____	14. Place the Aquathermia or heating device, if used, over the towel.	
____	____	____	15. Remove gloves and discard them appropriately. Perform hand hygiene, and remove additional PPE, if used.	
____	____	____	16. *Monitor the time the compress is in place to prevent burns and skin/tissue damage. Monitor the condition of the patient's skin and the patient's response at frequent intervals.*	
____	____	____	17. After the prescribed time for the treatment (up to 30 minutes), remove the external heating device (if used) and put on gloves.	
____	____	____	18. Carefully remove the compress while assessing the skin condition around the site and observing the patient's response to the heat application. Note any changes in the application area.	
____	____	____	19. Remove gloves. Place the patient in a comfortable position. Lower the bed. Dispose of any other supplies appropriately.	
____	____	____	20. Remove additional PPE, if used. Perform hand hygiene.	

Skill Checklists for Fundamentals of Nursing:
The Art and Science of Nursing Care, 7th edition

Name _____   Date _____

Unit _____   Position _____

Instructor/Evaluator: _____   Position _____

Excellent	Satisfactory	Needs Practice	SKILL 33-1 **Applying and Removing Antiembolism Stockings**	Comments
			Goal: The stockings will be applied and removed with minimal discomfort to the patient.	
——	——	——	1. Review the medical record and medical orders to determine the need for antiembolism stockings.	
——	——	——	2. Perform hand hygiene. Put on PPE, as indicated.	
——	——	——	3. Identify the patient. Explain what you are going to do and the rationale for use of elastic stockings.	
——	——	——	4. Close curtains around bed and close door to room if possible.	
——	——	——	5. Adjust the bed to a comfortable working height, usually elbow height of the caregiver (VISN 8, 2009).	
——	——	——	6. Assist patient to supine position. If patient has been sitting or walking, have him or her lie down with legs and feet well elevated for at least 15 minutes before applying stockings.	
——	——	——	7. Expose legs one at a time. Wash and dry legs, if necessary. Powder the leg lightly unless patient has a breathing problem, dry skin, or sensitivity to the powder. If the skin is dry, a lotion may be used. Powders and lotions are not recommended by some manufacturers; check the package material for manufacturer specifications.	
——	——	——	8. Stand at the foot of the bed. Place hand inside stocking and grasp heel area securely. Turn stocking inside out to the heel area, leaving the foot inside the stocking leg.	
——	——	——	9. With the heel pocket down, ease the foot of stocking over foot and heel. Check that patient's heel is centered in heel pocket of stocking.	
——	——	——	10. Using your fingers and thumbs, carefully grasp edge of stocking and pull it up smoothly over ankle and calf, toward the knee. Make sure it is distributed evenly.	
——	——	——	11. Pull forward slightly on toe section. If the stocking has a toe window, make sure it is properly positioned. Adjust if necessary to ensure material is smooth.	
——	——	——	12. If the stockings are knee-length, make sure each stocking top is 1 to 2 inches below the patella. Make sure the stocking does not roll down.	

SKILL 33-1

Applying and Removing Antiembolism Stockings *(Continued)*

Excellent	Satisfactory	Needs Practice		Comments

Excellent	Satisfactory	Needs Practice		Comments
——	——	——	13. If applying thigh-length stocking, continue the application. Flex the patient's leg. Stretch the stocking over the knee.	
——	——	——	14. Pull the stocking over the thigh until the top is 1 to 3 inches below the gluteal fold. Adjust the stocking as necessary to distribute the fabric evenly. Make sure the stocking does not roll down.	
——	——	——	15. Remove equipment and return patient to a position of comfort. Remove your gloves. Raise side rail and lower bed.	
——	——	——	16. Remove any other PPE, if used. Perform hand hygiene.	
			Removing Stockings	
——	——	——	17. To remove stocking, grasp top of stocking with your thumb and fingers and smoothly pull stocking off inside out to heel. Support foot and ease stocking over it.	

Skill Checklists for Fundamentals of Nursing:
The Art and Science of Nursing Care, 7th edition

Name _____   Date _____

Unit _____   Position _____

Instructor/Evaluator: _____   Position _____

Excellent	Satisfactory	Needs Practice	SKILL 33-2 **Assisting a Patient With Turning in Bed**	
			Goal: The activity takes place without injury to patient or nurse.	**Comments**
___	___	___	1. Review the physician's orders and nursing plan of care for patient activity. Identify any movement limitations and the ability of the patient to assist with turning. Consult patient-handling algorithm, if available, to plan appropriate approach to moving the patient.	
___	___	___	2. Gather any positioning aids or supports, if necessary.	
___	___	___	3. Perform hand hygiene. Put on PPE, as indicated.	
___	___	___	4. Identify the patient. Explain the procedure to the patient.	
___	___	___	5. Close the room door or curtains. Position at least one nurse on either side of the bed. Place pillows, wedges, or any other support to be used for positioning within easy reach. Place the bed at an appropriate and comfortable working height, usually elbow height of the caregiver (VISN 8, 2009). Lower both side rails.	
___	___	___	6. If not already in place, position a friction-reducing sheet under the patient.	
___	___	___	7. Using the friction-reducing sheet, move the patient to the edge of the bed, opposite the side to which he or she will be turned. Raise the side rails.	
___	___	___	8. If the patient is able, have the patient grasp the side rail on the side of the bed toward which they are turning. Alternately, place the patient's arms across his or her chest and cross his or her far leg over the leg nearest you.	
___	___	___	9. If available, activate the bed mechanism to inflate the side of the bed behind the patient's back.	
___	___	___	10. ***The nurse on the side of the bed toward which the patient is turning should stand opposite the patient's center with his or her feet spread about shoulder width and with one foot ahead of the other. Tighten your gluteal and abdominal muscles and flex your knees. Use your leg muscles to do the pulling. The other nurse should position his or her hands on the patient's shoulder and hip, assisting to roll the patient to the side. Instruct the patient to pull on the bed rail at the same time. Use the friction-reducing sheet to gently pull the patient over on his or her side.***	

SKILL 33-2

Assisting a Patient With Turning in Bed *(Continued)*

Excellent	Satisfactory	Needs Practice		Comments

			11. Use a pillow or other support behind the patient's back. Pull the shoulder blade forward and out from under the patient.	
			12. Make the patient comfortable and position in proper alignment, using pillows or other supports under the leg and arm as needed. Readjust the pillow under the patient's head. Elevate the head of the bed as needed for comfort.	
			13. *Place the bed in the lowest position, with the side rails up. Make sure the call bell and other necessary items are within easy reach.*	
			14. Clean transfer aids per facility policy, if not indicated for single patient use. Remove gloves and other PPE, if used. Perform hand hygiene.	

Skill Checklists for Fundamentals of Nursing:
The Art and Science of Nursing Care, 7th edition

Name _____ Date _____

Unit _____ Position _____

Instructor/Evaluator: _____ Position _____

SKILL 33-3

Moving a Patient Up in Bed With the Assistance of Another Nurse

Goal: The patient remains free from injury and maintains proper body alignment.

Excellent	Satisfactory	Needs Practice		Comments
____	____	____	1. Review the medical record and nursing plan of care for conditions that may influence the patient's ability to move or to be positioned. Assess for tubes, intravenous lines, incisions, or equipment that may alter the positioning procedure. Identify any movement limitations. Consult patient handling algorithm, if available, to plan appropriate approach to moving the patient.	
____	____	____	2. Perform hand hygiene and put on PPE, if indicated.	
____	____	____	3. Identify the patient. Explain the procedure to the patient.	
____	____	____	4. Close the room door or curtains. Place the bed at an appropriate and comfortable working height, usually elbow height of the caregiver (VISN 8, 2009). Adjust the head of the bed to a flat position or as low as the patient can tolerate. Placing the bed in slight Trendelenburg position aids movement, if the patient is able to tolerate it.	
____	____	____	5. Remove all pillows from under the patient. Leave one at the head of the bed, leaning upright against the headboard.	
____	____	____	6. Position at least one nurse on either side of the bed, and lower both side rails.	
____	____	____	7. If a friction-reducing sheet (or device) is not in place under the patient, place one under the patient's midsection.	
____	____	____	8. Ask the patient (if able) to bend his or her legs and put his or her feet flat on the bed to assist with the movement.	
____	____	____	9. Have the patient fold the arms across the chest. Have the patient (if able) lift the head with chin on chest.	
____	____	____	10. One nurse should be positioned on each side of the bed, at the patient's midsection with feet spread shoulder width apart and one foot slightly in front of the other.	
____	____	____	11. If available on bed, engage mechanism to make the bed surface firmer for repositioning.	
____	____	____	12. Grasp the friction-reducing sheet securely, close to the patient's body.	
____	____	____	13. Flex your knees and hips. Tighten your abdominal and gluteal muscles and keep your back straight.	

Excellent

Satisfactory

Needs Practice

SKILL 33-3

Moving a Patient Up in Bed With the Assistance of Another Nurse *(Continued)*

Comments

——	——	——	14. Shift your weight back and forth from your back leg to your front leg and count to three. On the count of three, move the patient up in bed. If possible, the patient can assist with the move by pushing with the legs. Repeat the process if necessary to get the patient to the right position.	
——	——	——	15. *Assist the patient to a comfortable position and readjust the pillows and supports as needed. Return bed surface to normal setting, if necessary. Raise the side rails. Place the bed in the lowest position.*	
——	——	——	16. Clean transfer aids per facility policy, if not indicated for single patient use. Remove gloves or other PPE, if used. Perform hand hygiene.	

Skill Checklists for Fundamentals of Nursing:
The Art and Science of Nursing Care, 7th edition

Name _____   Date _____

Unit _____   Position _____

Instructor/Evaluator: _____   Position _____

Excellent	Satisfactory	Needs Practice	SKILL 33-4
			## Transferring a Patient From the Bed to a Stretcher

Goal: The patient is transferred without injury to patient or nurse.   **Comments**

Excellent	Satisfactory	Needs Practice		Comments
——	——	——	1. Review the medical record and nursing plan of care for conditions that may influence the patient's ability to move or to be positioned. Assess for tubes, IV lines, incisions, or equipment that may alter the positioning procedure. Identify any movement limitations. Consult patient-handling algorithm, if available, to plan appropriate approach to moving the patient.	
——	——	——	2. Perform hand hygiene and put on PPE, if indicated.	
——	——	——	3. Identify the patient. Explain the procedure to the patient.	
——	——	——	4. Close the room door or curtains. Adjust the head of the bed to a flat position or as low as the patient can tolerate. Raise the bed to a height that is even with the transport stretcher (VISN 8, 2009). Lower the side rails, if in place.	
——	——	——	5. Place the bath blanket over the patient and remove the top covers from underneath.	
——	——	——	6. If a friction-reducing transfer sheet is not in place under the patient, place one under the patient's midsection. Have patient fold arms against chest and move chin to chest. Use the friction-reducing sheet to move the patient to the side of the bed where the stretcher will be placed. Alternately, place a lateral-assist device under the patient. Follow manufacturer's directions for use.	
——	——	——	7. Position the stretcher next to and parallel to the bed. *Lock the wheels on the stretcher and the bed.*	
——	——	——	8. The two nurses should stand on the stretcher side of the bed. The third nurse should stand on the side of the bed without the stretcher.	
——	——	——	9. Use the friction-reducing sheet to roll the patient away from the stretcher. Place the transfer board across the space between the stretcher and the bed, partially under the patient. Roll the patient onto his back, so he is partially on transfer board.	

SKILL 33-4

Transferring a Patient From the Bed to a Stretcher *(Continued)*

Excellent	Satisfactory	Needs Practice		Comments
___	___	___	10. The nurse on the side of the bed without the stretcher should grasp the friction-reducing sheet at the head and chest areas of the patient. One nurse on the stretcher side of the bed should grasp the friction-reducing sheet at the head and chest, and the other nurse at the chest and leg areas of the patient.	
___	___	___	11. *At a signal given by one of the nurses, have the nurses standing on the stretcher side of the bed pull the friction-reducing sheet. At the same time, the nurse (or nurses) on the other side push, transferring the patient's weight toward the transfer board, and pushing the patient from the bed to the stretcher.*	
___	___	___	12. Once the patient is transferred to the stretcher, remove the transfer board, and secure the patient until the side rails are raised. Raise the side rails. Ensure the patient's comfort. Cover the patient with blanket and remove the bath blanket from underneath. Leave the friction-reducing sheet in place for the return transfer.	
___	___	___	13. Clean transfer aids per facility policy, if not indicated for single patient use. Remove gloves and any other PPE, if used. Perform hand hygiene.	

Skill Checklists for Fundamentals of Nursing:
The Art and Science of Nursing Care, 7th edition

Name _____   Date _____

Unit _____   Position _____

Instructor/Evaluator: _____   Position _____

SKILL 33-5

Transferring a Patient From the Bed to a Chair

Goal: The transfer is accomplished without injury to patient or nurse and the patient remains free of any complications of immobility.

Excellent	Satisfactory	Needs Practice		Comments
____	____	____	1. Review the medical record and nursing plan of care for conditions that may influence the patient's ability to move or to be positioned. Assess for tubes, IV lines, incisions, or equipment that may alter the positioning procedure. Identify any movement limitations. Consult patient-handling algorithm, if available, to plan appropriate approach to moving the patient.	
____	____	____	2. Perform hand hygiene and put on PPE, as indicated.	
____	____	____	3. Identify the patient. Explain the procedure to the patient.	
____	____	____	4. If needed, move equipment to make room for the chair. Close the door or draw the curtains.	
____	____	____	5. Place the bed in the lowest position. Raise the head of the bed to a sitting position, or as high as the patient can tolerate.	
____	____	____	6. *Make sure the bed brakes are locked. Put the chair next to the bed. If available, lock the brakes of the chair. If the chair does not have brakes, brace the chair against a secure object.*	
____	____	____	7. Encourage the patient to make use of a stand-assist aid, either free-standing or attached to the side of the bed, if available, to move to the side of the bed and to a side-lying position, facing the side of the bed the patient will sit on.	
____	____	____	8. Lower the side rail if necessary and stand near the patient's hips. Stand with your legs shoulder width apart with one foot near the head of the bed, slightly in front of the other foot.	
____	____	____	9. Encourage the patient to make use of the stand-assist device. Assist the patient to sit up on the side of the bed; ask the patient to swing his or her legs over the side of the bed. At the same time, pivot on your back leg to lift the patient's trunk and shoulders. Keep your back straight; avoid twisting.	
____	____	____	10. *Stand in front of the patient, and assess for any balance problems or complaints of dizziness. Allow legs to dangle a few minutes before continuing.*	

Transferring a Patient From the Bed to a Chair *(Continued)*

Excellent	Satisfactory	Needs Practice		Comments
——	——	——	11. Assist the patient to put on a robe, as necessary, and non-skid footwear.	
——	——	——	12. Wrap the gait belt around the patient's waist, based on assessed need and facility policy.	
——	——	——	13. Stand facing the patient. Spread your feet about shoulder width apart and flex your hips and knees.	
——	——	——	14. Ask the patient to slide his or her buttocks to the edge of the bed until the feet touch the floor. Position yourself as close as possible to the patient, with your foot positioned on the outside of the patient's foot. If a second staff person is assisting, have him/her assume a similar position.	
——	——	——	15. Encourage the patient to make use of the stand-assist device. If necessary, have second staff person grasp gait belt on opposite side. Using the gait belt, assist the patient to stand. Rock back and forth while counting to three. *On the count of three, use your legs (not your back) to help raise the patient to a standing position.* If indicated, brace your front knee against the patient's weak extremity as he or she stands. Assess the patient's balance and leg strength. If the patient is weak or unsteady, return the patient to bed.	
——	——	——	16. Pivot on your back foot and assist the patient to turn until the patient feels the chair against his or her legs.	
——	——	——	17. Ask the patient to use an arm to steady himself or herself on the arm of the chair while slowly lowering to a sitting position. Continue to brace the patient's knees with your knees and hold the gait belt. Flex your hips and knees when helping the patient sit in the chair.	
——	——	——	18. Assess the patient's alignment in the chair. Remove gait belt, if desired. Depending on patient comfort, it could be left in place to use when returning to bed. Cover with a blanket if needed. Place the call bell close.	
——	——	——	19. Clean transfer aids per facility policy, if not indicated for single patient use. Remove gloves and any other PPE, if used. Perform hand hygiene.	

Skill Checklists for Fundamentals of Nursing:
The Art and Science of Nursing Care, 7th edition

Name _____ Date _____

Unit _____ Position _____

Instructor/Evaluator: _____ Position _____

SKILL 33-6

Providing Range-of-Motion Exercises

Excellent	Satisfactory	Needs Practice	**Goal:** The patient maintains joint mobility.	Comments
——	——	——	1. Review the physician's orders and nursing plan of care for patient activity. Identify any movement limitations.	
——	——	——	2. Perform hand hygiene and put on PPE, if indicated.	
——	——	——	3. Identify the patient. Explain the procedure to the patient.	
——	——	——	4. Close the room door or curtains. Place the bed at an appropriate and comfortable working height, usually elbow height of the caregiver (VISN 8, 2009). Adjust the head of the bed to a flat position or as low as the patient can tolerate.	
——	——	——	5. Stand on the side of the bed where the joints are to be exercised. Lower side rail on that side, if in place. Uncover only the limb to be used during the exercise.	
——	——	——	6. Perform the exercises slowly and gently, providing support by holding the areas proximal and distal to the joint. Repeat each exercise two to five times, moving each joint in a smooth and rhythmic manner. *Stop movement if the patient complains of pain or if you meet resistance.*	
——	——	——	7. While performing the exercises, begin at the head and move down one side of the body at a time. *Encourage the patient to do as many of these exercises by himself or herself as possible.*	
——	——	——	8. Move the chin down to rest on the chest. Return the head to a normal upright position. Tilt the head as far as possible toward each shoulder.	
——	——	——	9. Move the head from side to side, bringing the chin toward each shoulder.	
——	——	——	10. Start with the arm at the patient's side and lift the arm forward to above the head. Return the arm to the starting position at the side of the body.	
——	——	——	11. With the arm back at the patient's side, move the arm laterally to an upright position above the head, and then return to the original position. Move the arm across the body as far as possible.	

SKILL 33-6

Providing Range-of-Motion Exercises *(Continued)*

Excellent	Satisfactory	Needs Practice		Comments
——	——	——	12. Raise the arm at the side until the upper arm is in line with the shoulder. Bend the elbow at a 90-degree angle and move the forearm upward and downward, then return the arm to the side.	
——	——	——	13. Bend the elbow and move the lower arm and hand upward toward the shoulder. Return the lower arm and hand to the original position while straightening the elbow.	
——	——	——	14. Rotate the lower arm and hand so the palm is up. Rotate the lower arm and hand so the palm of the hand is down.	
——	——	——	15. Move the hand downward toward the inner aspect of the forearm. Return the hand to a neutral position even with the forearm. Then move the dorsal portion of the hand backward as far as possible.	
——	——	——	16. Bend the fingers to make a fist, and then straighten them out. Spread the fingers apart and return them back together. Touch the thumb to each finger on the hand.	
——	——	——	17. Extend the leg and lift it upward. Return the leg to the original position beside the other leg.	
——	——	——	18. Lift the leg laterally away from the patient's body. Return the leg back toward the other leg and try to extend it beyond the midline.	
——	——	——	19. Turn the foot and leg toward the other leg to rotate it internally. Turn the foot and leg outward away from the other leg to rotate it externally.	
——	——	——	20. Bend the leg and bring the heel toward the back of the leg. Return the leg to a straight position.	
——	——	——	21. At the ankle, move the foot up and back until the toes are upright. Move the foot with the toes pointing downward.	
——	——	——	22. Turn the sole of the foot toward the midline. Turn the sole of the foot outward.	
——	——	——	23. Curl the toes downward, and then straighten them out. Spread the toes apart and bring them together.	
——	——	——	24. Repeat these exercises on the other side of the body. Encourage the patient to do as many of these exercises by himself or herself as possible.	
——	——	——	25. *When finished, make sure the patient is comfortable, with the side rails up and the bed in the lowest position.*	
——	——	——	26. Remove gloves and any other PPE, if used. Perform hand hygiene.	

Skill Checklists for Fundamentals of Nursing:
The Art and Science of Nursing Care, 7th edition

Name _____ Date _____

Unit _____ Position _____

Instructor/Evaluator: _____ Position _____

SKILL 35-1

Giving a Back Massage

Goal: The patient reports increased comfort and decreased pain, and is relaxed.

Excellent	Satisfactory	Needs Practice		Comments
——	——	——	1. Perform hand hygiene and put on PPE, if indicated.	
——	——	——	2. Identify the patient.	
——	——	——	3. Offer a back massage to the patient and explain the procedure.	
——	——	——	4. Put on gloves, if indicated.	
——	——	——	5. Close room door and/or curtain.	
——	——	——	6. Assess the patient's pain, using an appropriate assessment tool and measurement scale.	
——	——	——	7. Raise bed to a comfortable working position, usually elbow height of the caregiver (VISN 8, 2009), and lower the side rail.	
——	——	——	8. Assist the patient to a comfortable position, preferably the prone or side-lying position. Remove the covers and move the patient's gown just enough to expose the patient's back from the shoulders to sacral area. Drape the patient as needed with the bath blanket.	
——	——	——	9. Warm the lubricant or lotion in the palm of your hand, or place the container in small basin of warm water. *During massage, observe the patient's skin for reddened or open areas. Pay particular attention to the skin over bony prominences.*	
——	——	——	10. Using light gliding strokes (*effleurage*), apply lotion to patient's shoulders, back, and sacral area.	
——	——	——	11. Place your hands beside each other at the base of the patient's spine and stroke upward to the shoulders and back downward to the buttocks in slow, continuous strokes. Continue for several minutes.	
——	——	——	12. Massage the patient's shoulder, entire back, areas over iliac crests, and sacrum with circular stroking motions. *Keep your hands in contact with the patient's skin.* Continue for several minutes, applying additional lotion as necessary.	
——	——	——	13. Knead the patient's skin by gently alternating grasping and compression motions (*pétrissage*).	
——	——	——	14. Complete the massage with additional long stroking movements that eventually become lighter in pressure.	

SKILL 35-1

Giving a Back Massage *(Continued)*

Excellent	Satisfactory	Needs Practice		Comments
——	——	——	15. Use the towel to pat the patient dry and to remove excess lotion.	
——	——	——	16. Remove gloves, if worn. Reposition patient gown and covers. Raise side rail and lower bed. Assist patient to a position of comfort.	
——	——	——	17. Remove additional PPE, if used. Perform hand hygiene.	
——	——	——	18. Evaluate the patient's response to interventions. Reassess level of discomfort or pain using original assessment tools. Reassess and alter plan of care as appropriate.	

Skill Checklists for Fundamentals of Nursing:
The Art and Science of Nursing Care, 7th edition

Name _____   Date _____

Unit _____   Position _____

Instructor/Evaluator: _____   Position _____

Skill 36-1
Inserting a Nasogastric (NG) Tube

Goal: The tube is passed into the patient's stomach without any complications.

Excellent	Satisfactory	Needs Practice		Comments
___	___	___	1. Verify the medical order for insertion of an NG tube.	
___	___	___	2. Perform hand hygiene and put on PPE, if indicated.	
___	___	___	3. Identify the patient.	
___	___	___	4. Explain the procedure to the patient and provide the rationale as to why the tube is needed. Discuss the associated discomforts that may be experienced and possible interventions that may allay this discomfort. Answer any questions, as needed.	
___	___	___	5. Gather equipment, including selection of the appropriate NG tube.	
___	___	___	6. Close the patient's bedside curtain or door. Raise bed to a comfortable working position, usually elbow height of the caregiver (VISN 8, 2009). Assist the patient to high Fowler's position or elevate the head of the bed 45 degrees if the patient is unable to maintain upright position. Drape chest with bath towel or disposable pad. Have emesis basin and tissues handy.	
___	___	___	7. *Measure the distance to insert tube by placing tip of tube at patient's nostril and extending to tip of earlobe and then to tip of xiphoid process.* Mark tube with an indelible marker.	
___	___	___	8. Put on gloves. Lubricate tip of tube (at least 2″–4″) with water-soluble lubricant. Apply topical anesthetic to nostril and oropharynx, as appropriate.	
___	___	___	9. After selecting the appropriate nostril, ask patient to slightly flex head back against the pillow. Gently insert the tube into the nostril while directing the tube upward and backward along the floor of the nose. Patient may gag when tube reaches pharynx. Provide tissues for tearing or watering of eyes. Offer comfort and reassurance to the patient.	

Skill 36-1

Inserting a Nasogastric (NG) Tube *(Continued)*

Excellent	Satisfactory	Needs Practice		Comments
——	——	——	10. When pharynx is reached, instruct patient to touch chin to chest. Encourage patient to sip water through a straw or swallow even if no fluids are permitted. Advance tube in downward and backward direction when patient swallows. Stop when patient breathes. *If gagging and coughing persist, stop advancing the tube and check placement of tube with tongue blade and flashlight.* If tube is curled, straighten the tube and attempt to advance again. Keep advancing tube until pen marking is reached. *Do not use force. Rotate tube if it meets resistance.*	
——	——	——	11. *Discontinue procedure and remove tube if there are signs of distress such as gasping, coughing, cyanosis, and inability to speak or hum.*	
——	——	——	12. Secure the tube loosely to the nose or cheek until it is determined that the tube is in the patient's stomach:	
——	——	——	a. Attach syringe to end of tube and aspirate a small amount of stomach contents.	
——	——	——	b. Measure the pH of aspirated fluid using pH paper or a meter. Place a drop of gastric secretions onto pH paper or place small amount in plastic cup and dip the pH paper into it. Within 30 seconds, compare the color on the paper with the chart supplied by the manufacturer.	
——	——	——	c. Visualize aspirated contents, checking for color and consistency.	
——	——	——	d. Obtain radiograph (x-ray) of placement of tube, based on facility policy (and ordered by physician).	
——	——	——	13. Apply skin barrier to tip and end of nose and allow to dry. Remove gloves and secure tube with a commercially prepared device (follow manufacturer's directions) or tape to patient's nose. To secure with tape:	
——	——	——	a. Cut a 4″ piece of tape and split bottom 2″ or use packaged nose tape for NG tubes.	
——	——	——	b. Place unsplit end over bridge of patient's nose.	
——	——	——	c. Wrap split ends under tubing and up and over onto nose. *Be careful not to pull tube too tightly against nose.*	
——	——	——	14. Put on gloves. Clamp tube and remove the syringe. Cap the tube or attach tube to suction according to the medical orders.	

Skill 36-1

Inserting a Nasogastric (NG) Tube *(Continued)*

Excellent	Satisfactory	Needs Practice		Comments
——	——	——	15. Measure length of exposed tube. Reinforce marking on tube at nostril with indelible ink. Ask the patient to turn their head to the side opposite the nostril the tube is inserted. Secure tube to patient's gown by using rubber band or tape and safety pin. For additional support, tube can be taped onto patient's cheek using a piece of tape. *If a double-lumen tube (e.g., Salem sump) is used, secure vent above stomach level.* Attach at shoulder level.	
——	——	——	16. Assist with or provide oral hygiene at 2- to 4-hour intervals. Lubricate the lips generously, clean nares, and lubricate, as needed. Offer analgesic throat lozenges or anesthetic spray for throat irritation if needed.	
——	——	——	17. Remove equipment and return patient to a position of comfort. Remove gloves. Raise side rail and lower bed.	
——	——	——	18. Remove additional PPE, if used. Perform hand hygiene.	

Skill Checklists for Fundamentals of Nursing:
The Art and Science of Nursing Care, 7th edition

Name _____   Date _____

Unit _____   Position _____

Instructor/Evaluator: _____   Position _____

SKILL 36-2

Administering a Tube Feeding

Goal: The patient receives the tube feeding without complaints of nausea or episodes of vomiting.

Excellent	Satisfactory	Needs Practice		Comments
___	___	___	1. Assemble equipment. Check amount, concentration, type, and frequency of tube feeding on patient's chart. Check expiration date of formula.	
___	___	___	2. Perform hand hygiene and put on PPE, if indicated.	
___	___	___	3. Identify the patient.	
___	___	___	4. Explain the procedure to the patient and why this intervention is needed. Answer any questions as needed.	
___	___	___	5. Assemble equipment on overbed table within reach.	
___	___	___	6. Close the patient's bedside curtain or door. Raise bed to a comfortable working position, usually elbow height of the caregiver (VISN 8, 2009). Perform key abdominal assessments as described above.	
___	___	___	7. *Position patient with head of bed elevated at least 30 to 45 degrees or as near normal position for eating as possible.*	
___	___	___	8. Put on gloves. Unpin tube from patient's gown. Verify the position of the marking on the tube at the nostril. Measure length of exposed tube and compare with the documented length.	
___	___	___	9. Attach syringe to end of tube and aspirate a small amount of stomach contents, as described in Skill 36-1.	
___	___	___	10. Check the pH as described in Skill 36-1.	
___	___	___	11. Visualize aspirated contents, checking for color and consistency.	
___	___	___	12. If it is not possible to aspirate contents; assessments to check placement are inconclusive; the exposed tube length has changed; or there are any other indications that the tube is not in place, check placement by x-ray.	
___	___	___	13. After multiple steps have been taken to ensure that the feeding tube is located in the stomach or small intestine, *aspirate all gastric contents with the syringe and measure to check for the residual amount of feeding in the stomach.* Return the residual based on facility policy. Proceed with feeding if amount of residual does not exceed agency policy or the limit indicated in the medical record.	

SKILL 36-2

Administering a Tube Feeding *(Continued)*

Excellent	Satisfactory	Needs Practice		Comments

14. Flush tube with 30 mL of water for irrigation. Disconnect syringe from tubing and cap end of tubing while preparing the formula feeding equipment. Remove gloves.

15. Put on gloves before preparing, assembling, and handling any part of the feeding system.

16. Administer feeding.

When Using a Feeding Bag (Open System)

a. Label bag and/or tubing with date and time. Hang bag on IV pole and adjust to about 12″ above the stomach. Clamp tubing.

b. Check the expiration date of the formula. Cleanse top of feeding container with a disinfectant before opening it. Pour formula into feeding bag and allow solution to run through tubing. Close clamp.

c. Attach feeding setup to feeding tube, open clamp, and regulate drip according to the medical order, or allow feeding to run in over 30 minutes.

d. *Add 30 to 60 mL (1–2 oz) of water for irrigation to feeding bag when feeding is almost completed and allow it to run through the tube.*

e. Clamp tubing immediately after water has been instilled. Disconnect **feeding setup** from feeding tube. Clamp tube and cover end with cap.

When Using a Large Syringe (Open System)

a. Remove plunger from 30- or 60-mL syringe.

b. Attach syringe to feeding tube, pour premeasured amount of tube feeding formula into syringe, open clamp, and allow food to enter tube. *Regulate rate, fast or slow, by height of the syringe. Do not push formula with syringe plunger.*

c. *Add 30 to 60 mL (1–2 oz) of water for irrigation to syringe when feeding is almost completed, and allow it to run through the tube.*

d. When syringe has emptied, hold syringe high and disconnect from tube. Clamp tube and cover end with cap.

Excellent	Satisfactory	Needs Practice	SKILL 36-2 **Administering a Tube Feeding** *(Continued)*	
				Comments
			When Using an Enteral Feeding Pump	
——	——	——	a. Close flow-regulator clamp on tubing and fill feeding bag with prescribed formula. Amount used depends on agency policy. Place label on container with patient's name, date, and time the feeding was hung.	
——	——	——	b. Hang feeding container on IV pole. *Allow solution to flow through tubing.*	
——	——	——	c. Connect to feeding pump following manufacturer's directions. Set rate. Maintain the patient in the upright position throughout the feeding. If the patient needs to temporarily lie flat, the feeding should be paused. The feeding may be resumed after the patient's position has been changed back to at least 30 to 45 degrees.	
——	——	——	d. *Check placement of tube and gastric residual every 4 to 6 hours.*	
——	——	——	17. Observe the patient's response during and after tube feeding and assess the abdomen at least once a shift.	
——	——	——	18. *Have patient remain in upright position for at least 1 hour after feeding.*	
——	——	——	19. Remove equipment and return patient to a position of comfort. Remove gloves. Raise side rail and lower bed.	
——	——	——	20. Put on gloves. Wash and clean equipment or replace according to agency policy. Remove gloves.	
——	——	——	21. Remove additional PPE, if used. Perform hand hygiene.	

Skill Checklists for Fundamentals of Nursing:
The Art and Science of Nursing Care, 7th edition

Name _____ Date _____

Unit _____ Position _____

Instructor/Evaluator: _____ Position _____

Excellent	Satisfactory	Needs Practice	SKILL 36-3 **Removing a Nasogastric Tube**	Comments
			Goal: The tube is removed with minimal discomfort to the patient, and the patient maintains an adequate nutritional intake.	
——	——	——	1. Check medical order for removal of NG tube.	
——	——	——	2. Perform hand hygiene and put on PPE, if indicated.	
——	——	——	3. Identify the patient.	
——	——	——	4. Explain the procedure to the patient and why this intervention is warranted. Describe that it will entail a quick few moments of discomfort. Perform key abdominal assessments as described above.	
——	——	——	5. Pull the patient's bedside curtain. Raise bed to a comfortable working position, usually elbow height of the caregiver (VISN 8, 2009). Assist the patient into a 30- to 45-degree position. Place towel or disposable pad across patient's chest. Give tissues and emesis basin to patient.	
——	——	——	6. Put on gloves. Discontinue suction and separate tube from suction. Unpin tube from patient's gown and carefully remove adhesive tape from patient's nose.	
——	——	——	7. Check placement (as outlined in Skill 36-1) and *attach syringe and flush with 10 mL of water or normal saline solution (optional) or clear with 30 to 50 mL of air.*	
——	——	——	8. *Clamp tube with fingers by doubling tube on itself. Instruct patient to take a deep breath and hold it. Quickly and carefully remove tube while patient holds breath.* Coil the tube in the disposable pad as you remove from the patient.	
——	——	——	9. Dispose of tube per agency policy. Remove gloves and place in bag. Perform hand hygiene.	
——	——	——	10. Offer mouth care to patient and facial tissue to blow nose. Lower the bed and assist the patient to a position of comfort, as needed.	
——	——	——	11. Remove equipment and raise side rail and lower bed.	
——	——	——	12. Put on gloves and measure the amount of nasogastric drainage in the collection device and record on output flow record, subtracting irrigant fluids if necessary. Add solidifying agent to nasogastric drainage according to hospital policy.	
——	——	——	13. Remove additional PPE, if used. Perform hand hygiene.	

Skill Checklists for Fundamentals of Nursing:
The Art and Science of Nursing Care, 7th edition

Name _____ Date _____

Unit _____ Position _____

Instructor/Evaluator: _____ Position _____

SKILL 36-4

Obtaining a Capillary Blood Sample for Glucose Testing

Excellent	Satisfactory	Needs Practice	**Goal:** Patient blood glucose levels are accurately monitored.	Comments
___	___	___	1. Check the patient's medical record or nursing plan of care for monitoring schedule. You may decide that additional testing is indicated based on nursing judgment and the patient's condition.	
___	___	___	2. Gather equipment.	
___	___	___	3. Perform hand hygiene and put on PPE, if indicated.	
___	___	___	4. Identify the patient. Explain procedure to patient and instruct patient about the need for monitoring blood glucose.	
___	___	___	5. Close curtains around bed and close door to room if possible.	
___	___	___	6. Turn the monitor on.	
___	___	___	7. Enter the patient's identification number, if required, according to facility policy.	
___	___	___	8. Put on nonsterile gloves.	
___	___	___	9. Prepare lancet using aseptic technique.	
___	___	___	10. Remove test strip from the vial. *Recap container immediately.* Test strips also come individually wrapped. *Check that code number for the strip matches code number on monitor screen.*	
___	___	___	11. Insert strip into the meter according to directions for that specific device.	
___	___	___	12. For adult, massage side of finger toward puncture site.	
___	___	___	13. *Have patient wash hands with soap and warm water and dry thoroughly. Alternately, cleanse the skin with an alcohol swab. Allow skin to dry completely.*	
___	___	___	14. Hold lancet perpendicular to skin and pierce site with lancet.	
___	___	___	15. Wipe away first drop of blood with gauze square or cotton ball, if recommended by manufacturer of monitor.	
___	___	___	16. Encourage bleeding by lowering hand, making use of gravity. Lightly stroke the finger, if necessary, until sufficient amount of blood has formed to cover the sample area on the strip, based on monitor requirements (check instructions for monitor). Take care not to squeeze the finger, not to squeeze at puncture site, or not to touch puncture site or blood.	

Excellent	Satisfactory	Needs Practice		Comments

SKILL 36-4

Obtaining a Capillary Blood Sample for Glucose Testing *(Continued)*

Excellent	Satisfactory	Needs Practice		Comments
___	___	___	17. Gently touch a drop of blood to pad to the test strip without smearing it.	
___	___	___	18. Press time button if directed by manufacturer.	
___	___	___	19. Apply pressure to puncture site with a cotton ball or dry gauze. *Do not use alcohol wipe.*	
___	___	___	20. Read blood glucose results and document appropriately at bedside. Inform patient of test result.	
___	___	___	21. Turn meter off, remove test strip and dispose of supplies appropriately. Place lancet in sharps container.	
___	___	___	22. Remove gloves and any other PPE, if used. Perform hand hygiene.	

Skill Checklists for Fundamentals of Nursing:
The Art and Science of Nursing Care, 7th edition

Name _____   Date _____

Unit _____   Position _____

Instructor/Evaluator: _____   Position _____

SKILL 37-1

Assessing Bladder Volume Using an Ultrasound Bladder Scanner

Goal: The volume of urine in the bladder is accurately measured.

Excellent	Satisfactory	Needs Practice		Comments
——	——	——	1. Review the patient's chart for any limitations in physical activity.	
——	——	——	2. Bring the bladder scanner and other necessary equipment to the bedside.	
——	——	——	3. Perform hand hygiene and put on PPE, if indicated.	
——	——	——	4. Identify the patient.	
——	——	——	5. Close curtains around bed and close door to room if possible. Discuss the procedure with the patient and assess patient's ability to assist with the procedure, as well as personal hygiene preferences.	
——	——	——	6. Adjust the bed to a comfortable working height, usually elbow height of the caregiver (VISN 8, 2009). Place the patient in a supine position. Drape patient. Stand on the patient's right side if you are right-handed, patient's left side if you are left-handed.	
——	——	——	7. Put on clean gloves.	
——	——	——	8. Press the "On" button. Wait until the device warms up. Press the "Scan" button to turn on the scanning screen.	
——	——	——	9. Press the appropriate gender button. The appropriate icon for male or female will appear on the screen.	
——	——	——	10. Clean the scanner head with the appropriate cleaner.	
——	——	——	11. *Gently palpate the patient's symphysis pubis. Place a generous amount of ultrasound gel or gel pad midline on the patient's abdomen, about 1" to 1 1/2" above the symphysis pubis (anterior midline junction of pubic bones).*	
——	——	——	12. *Place the scanner head on the gel or gel pad, with the directional icon on the scanner head toward the patient's head. Aim the scanner head toward the bladder (point the scanner head slightly downward toward the coccyx) (Patraca, 2005). Press and release the "Scan" button.*	
——	——	——	13. Observe the image on the scanner screen. *Adjust the scanner head to center the bladder image on the crossbars.*	

Excellent	Satisfactory	Needs Practice		Comments
——	——	——	14. Press and hold the "Done" button until it beeps. Read the volume measurement on the screen. Print the results, if required, by pressing "Print."	
——	——	——	15. Use a washcloth or paper towel to remove remaining gel from the patient's skin. Alternately, gently remove gel pad from patient's skin. Return the patient to a comfortable position. Remove your gloves and ensure that the patient is covered.	
——	——	——	16. Lower bed height and adjust head of bed to a comfortable position. Reattach call bell if necessary.	
——	——	——	17. Remove additional PPE, if used. Perform hand hygiene.	

Skill Checklists for Fundamentals of Nursing:
The Art and Science of Nursing Care, 7th edition

Name _____ Date _____

Unit _____ Position _____

Instructor/Evaluator: _____ Position _____

SKILL 37-2

Assisting With the Use of a Bedpan

Excellent	Satisfactory	Needs Practice	**Goal:** The patient is able to void with assistance.	Comments
___	___	___	1. Review the patient's chart for any limitations in physical activity.	
___	___	___	2. Bring bedpan and other necessary equipment to the bedside stand or overbed table.	
___	___	___	3. Perform hand hygiene and put on PPE, if indicated.	
___	___	___	4. Identify the patient.	
___	___	___	5. Close curtains around bed and close door to room if possible. Discuss the procedure with the patient and assess the patient's ability to assist with the procedure, as well as personal hygiene preferences.	
___	___	___	6. Unless contraindicated, apply powder to the rim of the bedpan. Place bedpan and cover on chair next to bed. Put on gloves.	
___	___	___	7. Adjust bed to comfortable working height, usually elbow height of the caregiver (VISN 8, 2009). Place the patient in a supine position, with the head of the bed elevated about 30 degrees, unless contraindicated.	
___	___	___	8. Fold top linen back just enough to allow placement of bedpan. If there is no waterproof pad on the bed and time allows, consider placing a waterproof pad under patient's buttocks before placing bedpan.	
___	___	___	9. Ask the patient to bend the knees. Have the patient lift his or her hips upward. Assist patient, if necessary, by placing your hand that is closest to the patient palm up, under the lower back, and assist with lifting. Slip the bedpan into place with other hand.	
___	___	___	10. *Ensure that bedpan is in proper position and patient's buttocks are resting on the rounded shelf of the regular bedpan or the shallow rim of the fracture bedpan.*	
___	___	___	11. Raise head of bed as near to sitting position as tolerated, unless contraindicated. Cover the patient with bed linens.	
___	___	___	12. *Place call bell and toilet tissue within easy reach. Place the bed in the lowest position.* Leave patient if it is safe to do so. Use side rails appropriately.	

SKILL 37-2

Assisting With the Use of a Bedpan *(Continued)*

Excellent	Satisfactory	Needs Practice		Comments
——	——	——	13. Remove gloves and additional PPE, if used. Perform hand hygiene.	

Removing the Bedpan

Excellent	Satisfactory	Needs Practice		Comments
——	——	——	14. Perform hand hygiene and put on gloves and additional PPE, as indicated. Adjust bed to comfortable working height, usually elbow height of the caregiver (VISN 8, 2009). Have a receptacle, such as plastic trash bag, handy for discarding tissue.	
——	——	——	15. Lower the head of the bed, if necessary, to about 30 degrees. Remove bedpan in the same manner in which it was offered, being careful to hold it steady. Ask the patient to bend the knees and lift the buttocks up from the bedpan. Assist patient, if necessary, by placing your hand that is closest to the patient palm up, under the lower back, and assist with lifting. Place the bedpan on the bedside chair and cover it.	
——	——	——	16. If patient needs assistance with hygiene, wrap tissue around the hand several times, and wipe patient clean, using one stroke from the pubic area toward the anal area. Discard tissue, and use more until patient is clean. Place patient on his or her side and spread buttocks to clean anal area.	
——	——	——	17. Do not place toilet tissue in the bedpan if a specimen is required or if output is being recorded. Place toilet tissue in appropriate receptacle.	
——	——	——	18. Return the patient to a comfortable position. Make sure the linens under the patient are dry. Replace or remove pad under the patient as necessary. Remove your gloves and ensure that the patient is covered.	
——	——	——	19. Raise side rail. Lower bed height and adjust head of bed to a comfortable position. Reattach call bell.	
——	——	——	20. Offer patient supplies to wash and dry his or her hands, assisting as necessary.	
——	——	——	21. Put on clean gloves. Empty and clean the bedpan, measuring urine in graduated container, as necessary. Discard trash receptacle with used toilet paper per facility policy.	
——	——	——	22. Remove additional PPE, if used. Perform hand hygiene.	

Skill Checklists for Fundamentals of Nursing:
The Art and Science of Nursing Care, 7th edition

Name _____ Date _____

Unit _____ Position _____

Instructor/Evaluator: _____ Position _____

Excellent	Satisfactory	Needs Practice	SKILL 37-3 **Assisting With the Use of a Urinal**	Comments
			Goal: The patient is able to void with assistance.	
___	___	___	1. Review the patient's chart for any limitations in physical activity.	
___	___	___	2. Bring urinal and other necessary equipment to the bedside stand or overbed table.	
___	___	___	3. Perform hand hygiene and put on PPE, if indicated.	
___	___	___	4. Identify the patient.	
___	___	___	5. Close the curtains around the bed and close the door to the room if possible. Discuss procedure with patient and assess the patient's ability to assist with the procedure, as well as personal hygiene preferences.	
___	___	___	6. Put on gloves.	
___	___	___	7. Assist the patient to an appropriate position as necessary: standing at the bedside, lying on one side or back, sitting in bed with the head elevated, or sitting on the side of the bed.	
___	___	___	8. If the patient remains in the bed, fold the linens just enough to allow for proper placement of the urinal.	
___	___	___	9. If the patient is not standing, have him spread his legs slightly. *Hold the urinal close to the penis and position the penis completely within the urinal. Keep the bottom of the urinal lower than the penis. If necessary, assist the patient to hold the urinal in place.*	
___	___	___	10. Cover the patient with the bed linens.	
___	___	___	11. Place call bell and toilet tissue within easy reach. Have a receptacle, such as plastic trash bag, handy for discarding tissue. Ensure the bed is in the lowest position. Leave patient if it is safe to do so. Use side rails appropriately.	
___	___	___	12. Remove gloves and additional PPE, if used. Perform hand hygiene.	
			Removing the Urinal	
___	___	___	13. Perform hand hygiene. Put on gloves and additional PPE, as indicated.	

Assisting With the Use of a Urinal *(Continued)*

Excellent	Satisfactory	Needs Practice		Comments
——	——	——	14. Pull back the patient's bed linens just enough to remove the urinal. Remove the urinal. Cover the open end of the urinal. Place on the bedside chair. If patient needs assistance with hygiene, wrap tissue around the hand several times, and wipe patient clean. Place tissue in receptacle.	
——	——	——	15. Return the patient to a comfortable position. Make sure the linens under the patient are dry. Remove your gloves and ensure that the patient is covered.	
——	——	——	16. Ensure patient call bell is in reach.	
——	——	——	17. Offer patient supplies to wash and dry his hands, assisting as necessary.	
——	——	——	18. Put on clean gloves. Empty and clean the urinal, measuring urine in graduated container, as necessary. Discard trash receptacle with used toilet paper per facility policy.	
——	——	——	19. Remove gloves and additional PPE, if used and perform hand hygiene.	

Skill Checklists for Fundamentals of Nursing:
The Art and Science of Nursing Care, 7th edition

Name _____ Date _____

Unit _____ Position _____

Instructor/Evaluator: _____ Position _____

Excellent	Satisfactory	Needs Practice	SKILL 37-4 **Applying an External Condom Catheter**	Comments
			Goal: The patient's urinary elimination will be maintained, with a urine output of at least 30 mL/hour, and the bladder is not distended.	
___	___	___	1. Bring necessary equipment to the bedside.	
___	___	___	2. Perform hand hygiene and put on PPE, if indicated.	
___	___	___	3. Identify the patient.	
___	___	___	4. Close curtains around bed and close door to room if possible. Discuss procedure with patient. Ask the patient if he has any allergies, especially to latex.	
___	___	___	5. Adjust bed to comfortable working height, usually elbow height of the caregiver (VISN 8, 2009). Stand on the patient's right side if you are right-handed, patient's left side if you are left-handed.	
___	___	___	6. Prepare urinary drainage setup or reusable leg bag for attachment to condom sheath.	
___	___	___	7. Position patient on his back with thighs slightly apart. Drape patient so that only the area around the penis is exposed. Slide waterproof pad under patient.	
___	___	___	8. Put on disposable gloves. Trim any long pubic hair that is in contact with penis.	
___	___	___	9. Clean the genital area with washcloth, skin cleanser, and warm water. If patient is uncircumcised, retract foreskin and clean glans of penis. Replace foreskin. Clean the tip of the penis first, moving the washcloth in a circular motion from the meatus outward. Wash the shaft of the penis using downward strokes toward the pubic area. Rinse and dry. Remove gloves. Perform hand hygiene again.	
___	___	___	10. Apply skin protectant to penis and allow to dry.	
___	___	___	11. Roll condom sheath outward onto itself. Grasp penis firmly with nondominant hand. *Apply condom sheath by rolling it onto penis with dominant hand. Leave 1" to 2" (2.5–5 cm) of space between tip of penis and end of condom sheath.*	
___	___	___	12. *Apply pressure to sheath at the base of penis for 10 to 15 seconds.*	
___	___	___	13. Connect condom sheath to drainage setup. Avoid kinking or twisting drainage tubing.	

SKILL 37-4

Applying an External Condom Catheter *(Continued)*

Excellent	Satisfactory	Needs Practice		Comments
——	——	——	14. Remove gloves. Secure drainage tubing to the patient's inner thigh with Velcro leg strap or tape. Leave some slack in tubing for leg movement.	
——	——	——	15. Assist the patient to a comfortable position. Cover the patient with bed linens. Place the bed in the lowest position.	
——	——	——	16. Secure drainage bag below the level of the bladder. Check that drainage tubing is not kinked and that movement of side rails does not interfere with the drainage bag.	
——	——	——	17. Remove equipment. Remove gloves and additional PPE, if used. Perform hand hygiene.	

Skill Checklists for Fundamentals of Nursing:
The Art and Science of Nursing Care, 7th edition

Name _____ Date _____

Unit _____ Position _____

Instructor/Evaluator: _____ Position _____

SKILL 37-5

Catheterizing the Female Urinary Bladder

Goal: The patient's urinary elimination is maintained, with a urine output of at least 30 mL/hour, and the patient's bladder is not distended.

Excellent	Satisfactory	Needs Practice		Comments
___	___	___	1. Review the patient's chart for any limitations in physical activity. Confirm the medical order for indwelling catheter insertion.	
___	___	___	2. Bring the catheter kit and other necessary equipment to the bedside. Obtain assistance from another staff member, if necessary.	
___	___	___	3. Perform hand hygiene and put on PPE, if indicated.	
___	___	___	4. Identify the patient.	
___	___	___	5. Close curtains around bed and close door to room if possible. Discuss procedure with the patient and assess patient's ability to assist with the procedure. Ask the patient if she has any allergies, especially to latex or iodine.	
___	___	___	6. Provide good lighting. Artificial light is recommended (use of a flashlight requires an assistant to hold and position it). Place a trash receptacle within easy reach.	
___	___	___	7. Adjust the bed to a comfortable working height, usually elbow height of the caregiver (VISN 8, 2009). Stand on the patient's right side if you are right-handed, patient's left side if you are left-handed.	
___	___	___	8. Assist the patient to a dorsal recumbent position with knees flexed, feet about 2 feet apart, with her legs abducted. Drape patient. Alternately, the Sims', or lateral, position can be used. Place the patient's buttocks near the edge of the bed with her shoulders at the opposite edge and her knees drawn toward her chest. Allow the patient to lie on either side, depending on which position is easiest for the nurse and best for the patient's comfort. Slide waterproof pad under patient.	
___	___	___	9. Put on clean gloves. Clean the perineal area with washcloth, skin cleanser, and warm water, using a different corner of the washcloth with each stroke. Wipe from above orifice downward toward sacrum (front to back). Rinse and dry. Remove gloves. Perform hand hygiene again.	
___	___	___	10. Prepare urine drainage setup if a separate urine collection system is to be used. Secure to bed frame according to manufacturer's directions.	

Catheterizing the Female Urinary Bladder *(Continued)*

Excellent	Satisfactory	Needs Practice		Comments

11. Open sterile catheterization tray on a clean overbed table using sterile technique.

12. Put on sterile gloves. Grasp upper corners of drape and unfold drape without touching unsterile areas. Fold back a corner on each side to make a cuff over gloved hands. Ask patient to lift her buttocks and slide sterile drape under her with gloves protected by cuff.

13. Based on facility policy, position the fenestrated sterile drape. Place a fenestrated sterile drape over the perineal area, exposing the labia.

14. Place sterile tray on drape between patient's thighs.

15. Open all the supplies. Fluff cotton balls in tray before pouring antiseptic solution over them. Alternately, open package of antiseptic swabs. Open specimen container if specimen is to be obtained.

16. Lubricate 1″ to 2″ of catheter tip.

17. With thumb and one finger of nondominant hand, spread labia and identify meatus. *Be prepared to maintain separation of labia with one hand until catheter is inserted and urine is flowing well and continuously.* If the patient is in the side-lying position, lift the upper buttock and labia to expose the urinary meatus.

18. Use the dominant hand to pick up a cotton ball or antiseptic swab. *Clean one labial fold, top to bottom (from above the meatus down toward the rectum), then discard the cotton ball. Using a new cotton ball/swab for each stroke, continue to clean the other labial fold, then directly over the meatus.*

19. With your uncontaminated, dominant hand, place drainage end of catheter in receptacle. If the catheter is preattached to sterile tubing and drainage container (closed drainage system), position catheter and setup within easy reach on sterile field. Ensure that clamp on drainage bag is closed.

Catheterizing the Female Urinary Bladder *(Continued)*

Excellent	Satisfactory	Needs Practice		Comments
——	——	——	20. *Using your dominant hand, hold the catheter 2" to 3" from the tip and insert slowly into the urethra. Advance the catheter until there is a return of urine (approximately 2" to 3" [4.8–7.2 cm]). Once urine drains, advance catheter another 2" to 3" (4.8–7.2 cm). Do not force catheter through urethra into bladder.* Ask patient to breathe deeply, and rotate catheter gently if slight resistance is met as catheter reaches external sphincter.	
——	——	——	21. Hold the catheter securely at the meatus with your nondominant hand. Use your dominant hand to inflate the catheter balloon. Inject entire volume of sterile water supplied in prefilled syringe.	
——	——	——	22. Pull gently on catheter after balloon is inflated to feel resistance.	
——	——	——	23. Attach catheter to drainage system if not already preattached.	
——	——	——	24. Remove equipment and dispose of it according to facility policy. Discard syringe in sharps container. Wash and dry the perineal area, as needed.	
——	——	——	25. Remove gloves. *Secure catheter tubing to the patient's inner thigh with Velcro leg strap or tape.* Leave some slack in catheter for leg movement.	
——	——	——	26. Assist the patient to a comfortable position. Cover the patient with bed linens. Place the bed in the lowest position.	
——	——	——	27. Secure drainage bag below the level of the bladder. Check that drainage tubing is not kinked and that movement of side rails does not interfere with catheter or drainage bag.	
——	——	——	28. Put on clean gloves. Obtain urine specimen immediately, if needed, from drainage bag. Label specimen. Send urine specimen to the laboratory promptly or refrigerate it.	
——	——	——	29. Remove gloves and additional PPE, if used. Perform hand hygiene.	

Name _____   Date _____

Unit _____   Position _____

Instructor/Evaluator: _____   Position _____

SKILL 37-6
Catheterizing the Male Urinary Bladder

Goal: The patient's urinary elimination is maintained, with a urine output of at least 30 mL/hour, and the patient's bladder is not distended.

Excellent	Satisfactory	Needs Practice		Comments
____	____	____	1. Review chart for any limitations in physical activity. Confirm the medical order for indwelling catheter insertion.	
____	____	____	2. Bring catheter kit and other necessary equipment to the bedside. Obtain assistance from another staff member, if necessary.	
____	____	____	3. Perform hand hygiene and put on PPE, if indicated.	
____	____	____	4. Identify the patient.	
____	____	____	5. Close curtains around bed and close door to room if possible. Discuss the procedure with the patient and assess patient's ability to assist with the procedure. Ask the patient if he has any allergies, especially to latex or iodine.	
____	____	____	6. Provide good lighting. Artificial light is recommended (use of a flashlight requires an assistant to hold and position it). Place a trash receptacle within easy reach.	
____	____	____	7. Adjust the bed to a comfortable working height, usually elbow height of the caregiver (VISN 8, 2009). Stand on the patient's right side if you are right-handed, patient's left side if you are left-handed.	
____	____	____	8. Position patient on his back with thighs slightly apart. Drape patient so that only the area around the penis is exposed. Slide waterproof pad under patient.	
____	____	____	9. Put on clean gloves. Clean the genital area with washcloth, skin cleanser, and warm water. Clean the tip of the penis first, moving the washcloth in a circular motion from the meatus outward. Wash the shaft of the penis using downward strokes toward the pubic area. Rinse and dry. Remove gloves. Perform hand hygiene again.	
____	____	____	10. Prepare urine drainage setup if a separate urine collection system is to be used. Secure to bed frame according to manufacturer's directions.	
____	____	____	11. Open sterile catheterization tray on a clean overbed table, using sterile technique.	
____	____	____	12. Put on sterile gloves. Open sterile drape and place on patient's thighs. Place fenestrated drape with opening over penis.	

Excellent	Satisfactory	Needs Practice	SKILL 37-6 **Catheterizing the Male Urinary Bladder** *(Continued)*	Comments
____	____	____	13. Place catheter set on or next to patient's legs on sterile drape.	
____	____	____	14. Open all the supplies. Fluff cotton balls in tray before pouring antiseptic solution over them. Alternately, open package of antiseptic swabs. Open specimen container if specimen is to be obtained. Remove cap from syringe pre-filled with lubricant.	
____	____	____	15. Place drainage end of catheter in receptacle. If the catheter is preattached to sterile tubing and drainage container (closed drainage system), position catheter and setup within easy reach on sterile field. Ensure that clamp on drainage bag is closed.	
____	____	____	16. Lift penis with nondominant hand. Retract foreskin in uncircumcised patient. *Be prepared to keep this hand in this position until catheter is inserted and urine is flowing well and continuously. Using the dominant hand and the forceps, pick up a cotton ball or antiseptic swab. Using a circular motion, clean the penis, moving from the meatus down the glans of the penis. Repeat this cleansing motion two more times, using a new cotton ball/swab each time. Discard each cotton ball/swab after one use.*	
____	____	____	17. Hold penis with slight upward tension and perpendicular to patient's body. Use the dominant hand to pick up the lubricant syringe. *Gently insert tip of syringe with lubricant into urethra and instill the 10 mL of lubricant* (SUNA, 2005c).	
____	____	____	18. Use the dominant hand to pick up the catheter and hold it an inch or two from the tip. Ask patient to bear down as if voiding. *Insert catheter tip into meatus. Ask the patient to take deep breaths. Advance the catheter to the bifurcation or "Y" level of the ports. Do not use force to introduce catheter.* If catheter resists entry, ask patient to breathe deeply and rotate catheter slightly.	
____	____	____	19. Hold the catheter securely at the meatus with your nondominant hand. Use your dominant hand to inflate the catheter balloon. *Inject entire volume of sterile water supplied in prefilled syringe. Once balloon is inflated, catheter may be gently pulled back into place. Replace foreskin over catheter.* Lower penis.	
____	____	____	20. Pull gently on catheter after balloon is inflated to feel resistance.	
____	____	____	21. Attach catheter to drainage system, if necessary.	

SKILL 37-6

Catheterizing the Male Urinary Bladder *(Continued)*

Excellent	Satisfactory	Needs Practice		Comments
——	——	——	22. Remove equipment and dispose of according to facility policy. Discard syringe in sharps container. Wash and dry the perineal area as needed.	
——	——	——	23. Remove gloves. Secure catheter tubing to the patient's inner thigh or lower abdomen (with the penis directed toward the patient's chest) with Velcro leg strap or tape. Leave some slack in catheter for leg movement.	
——	——	——	24. Assist the patient to a comfortable position. Cover the patient with bed linens. Place the bed in the lowest position.	
——	——	——	25. Secure drainage bag below the level of the bladder. Check that drainage tubing is not kinked and that movement of side rails does not interfere with catheter or drainage bag.	
——	——	——	26. Put on clean gloves. Obtain urine specimen immediately, if needed, from drainage bag. Label specimen. Send urine specimen to the laboratory promptly or refrigerate it.	
——	——	——	27. Remove gloves and additional PPE, if used. Perform hand hygiene.	

Skill Checklists for Fundamentals of Nursing:
The Art and Science of Nursing Care, 7th edition

Name _____   Date _____

Unit _____   Position _____

Instructor/Evaluator: _____   Position _____

SKILL 37-7
Performing Intermittent Closed Catheter Irrigation

Excellent	Satisfactory	Needs Practice		Comments
			Goal: The patient exhibits the free flow of urine through the catheter.	
——	——	——	1. Confirm the order for catheter irrigation in the medical record.	
——	——	——	2. Bring necessary equipment to the bedside.	
——	——	——	3. Perform hand hygiene and put on PPE, if indicated.	
——	——	——	4. Identify the patient.	
——	——	——	5. Close curtains around bed and close door to room if possible. Discuss procedure with patient.	
——	——	——	6. Adjust bed to comfortable working height, usually elbow height of the caregiver (VISN 8, 2009).	
——	——	——	7. Put on gloves. Empty the catheter drainage bag and measure the amount of urine, noting the amount and characteristics of the urine. Remove gloves.	
——	——	——	8. Assist patient to comfortable position and expose access port on catheter setup. Place waterproof pad under catheter and aspiration port. Remove catheter from device or tape anchoring catheter to the patient.	
——	——	——	9. Open supplies, using aseptic technique. Pour sterile solution into sterile basin. Aspirate the prescribed amount of irrigant (usually 30–60 mL) into sterile syringe. Put on gloves.	
——	——	——	10. *Cleanse the access port on catheter with antimicrobial swab.*	
——	——	——	11. Clamp or fold catheter tubing below the access port.	
——	——	——	12. Attach the syringe to the access port on catheter using a twisting motion. *Gently instill solution into catheter.*	
——	——	——	13. Remove syringe from access port. *Unclamp or unfold tubing and allow irrigant and urine to flow into the drainage bag.* Repeat procedure as necessary.	
——	——	——	14. Remove gloves. Secure catheter tubing to the patient's inner thigh or lower abdomen (if a male patient) with anchoring device or tape. Leave some slack in catheter for leg movement.	
——	——	——	15. Assist the patient to a comfortable position. Cover the patient with bed linens. Place the bed in the lowest position.	

Performing Intermittent Closed Catheter Irrigation *(Continued)*

Excellent	Satisfactory	Needs Practice		Comments
——	——	——	16. Secure drainage bag below the level of the bladder. Check that drainage tubing is not kinked and that movement of side rails does not interfere with catheter or drainage bag.	
——	——	——	17. Remove equipment and discard syringe in appropriate receptacle. Remove gloves and additional PPE, if used. Perform hand hygiene.	
——	——	——	18. Assess patient's response to procedure and quality and amount of drainage after the irrigation.	

Skill Checklists for Fundamentals of Nursing:
The Art and Science of Nursing Care, 7th edition

Name _____ Date _____

Unit _____ Position _____

Instructor/Evaluator: _____ Position _____

SKILL 37-8

Administering a Continuous Closed Bladder Irrigation

Goal: The patient exhibits free-flowing urine through the catheter.

Excellent	Satisfactory	Needs Practice		Comments
___	___	___	1. Confirm the order for catheter irrigation in the medical record. Calculate the drip rate via gravity infusion for prescribed infusion rate.	
___	___	___	2. Bring necessary equipment to the bedside.	
___	___	___	3. Perform hand hygiene and put on PPE, if indicated.	
___	___	___	4. Identify the patient.	
___	___	___	5. Close curtains around the bed and close the door to the room if possible. Discuss the procedure with patient.	
___	___	___	6. Adjust bed to comfortable working height, usually elbow height of the caregiver (VISN 8, 2009).	
___	___	___	7. Empty the catheter drainage bag and measure the amount of urine, noting the amount and characteristics of the urine.	
___	___	___	8. Assist patient to comfortable position and expose the irrigation port on the catheter setup. Place waterproof pad under catheter and aspiration port.	
___	___	___	9. Prepare sterile irrigation bag for use as directed by manufacturer. Clearly label the solution as "Bladder Irrigant." Include the date and time on the label. Hang bag on IV pole 2 1/2′ to 3′ above level of patient's bladder. Secure tubing clamp and insert sterile tubing with drip chamber to container using aseptic technique. Release clamp and remove protective cover on end of tubing without contaminating it. Allow solution to flush tubing and remove air. Clamp tubing and replace end cover.	
___	___	___	10. Put on gloves. *Cleanse the irrigation port on the catheter with an alcohol swab. Using aseptic technique, attach irrigation tubing to irrigation port of three-way indwelling catheter.*	
___	___	___	11. Check the drainage tubing to make sure clamp, if present, is open.	
___	___	___	12. *Release clamp on irrigation tubing and regulate flow at determined drip rate, according to the ordered rate.* If the bladder irrigation is to be done with a medicated solution, use an electronic infusion device to regulate the flow.	

Administering a Continuous Closed Bladder Irrigation *(Continued)*

Excellent	Satisfactory	Needs Practice		Comments
⎯	⎯	⎯	13. Remove gloves. Assist the patient to a comfortable position. Cover the patient with bed linens. Place the bed in the lowest position.	
⎯	⎯	⎯	14. Assess patient's response to procedure and quality and amount of drainage.	
⎯	⎯	⎯	15. Remove equipment. Remove gloves and additional PPE, if used. Perform hand hygiene.	
⎯	⎯	⎯	16. As irrigation fluid container nears empty, clamp the administration tubing. Do not allow drip chamber to empty. Disconnect empty bag and attach a new full irrigation solution bag.	
⎯	⎯	⎯	17. Put on gloves and empty drainage collection bag as each new container is hung and recorded.	

Skill Checklists for Fundamentals of Nursing:
The Art and Science of Nursing Care, 7th edition

Name _____   Date _____

Unit _____   Position _____

Instructor/Evaluator: _____   Position _____

Excellent	Satisfactory	Needs Practice	SKILL 37-9 **Emptying and Changing a Stoma Appliance on an Ileal Conduit**	Comments
			Goal: The stoma appliance is applied correctly to the skin to allow urine to drain freely.	
——	——	——	1. Bring necessary equipment to the bedside stand or overbed table.	
——	——	——	2. Perform hand hygiene and put on PPE, if indicated.	
——	——	——	3. Identify the patient.	
——	——	——	4. Close curtains around bed and close door to room if possible. Explain what you are going to do and why you are going to do it to the patient. Encourage patient to observe or participate if possible.	
——	——	——	5. Assist patient to a comfortable sitting or lying position in bed or a standing or sitting position in the bathroom. If the patient is in bed, adjust the bed to a comfortable working height, usually elbow height of the caregiver (VISN 8, 2009). Place waterproof pad under the patient at the stoma site.	
			Emptying the Appliance	
——	——	——	6. Put on gloves. Hold end of appliance over a bedpan, toilet, or measuring device. Remove the end cap from the spout. Open spout and empty contents into the bedpan, toilet, or measuring device.	
——	——	——	7. Close the spout. Wipe the spout with toilet tissue. Replace the cap.	
——	——	——	8. Remove equipment. Remove gloves. Assist patient to comfortable position.	
——	——	——	9. If appliance is not to be changed, place bed in lowest position. Remove additional PPE, if used. Perform hand hygiene.	
			Changing the Appliance	
——	——	——	10. Place a disposable waterproof pad on the overbed table or other work area. Set up the washbasin with warm water and the rest of the supplies. Place a trash bag within reach.	
——	——	——	11. Put on clean gloves. Place waterproof pad under the patient at the stoma site. Empty the appliance if necessary as described in Steps 6 to 8.	

Excellent	Satisfactory	Needs Practice		Comments

Emptying and Changing a Stoma Appliance on an Ileal Conduit *(Continued)*

Excellent	Satisfactory	Needs Practice		Comments
——	——	——	12. Gently remove appliance faceplate from skin by pushing skin from appliance rather than pulling appliance from skin. Start at the top of the appliance, while keeping the skin taut. Apply a silicone-based adhesive remover by spraying or wiping with the remover wipe. Push the skin from the appliance rather than pulling the appliance from the skin.	
——	——	——	13. Place the appliance in the trash bag, if disposable. If reusable, set aside to wash in lukewarm soap and water and allow to air dry after the new appliance is in place.	
——	——	——	14. Clean skin around stoma with mild soap and water or a cleansing agent and a washcloth. Remove all old adhesive from skin; additional adhesive remover may be used. Do not apply lotion to peristomal area.	
——	——	——	15. Gently pat area dry. *Make sure skin around stoma is thoroughly dry.* Assess stoma and condition of surrounding skin.	
——	——	——	16. Place one or two gauze squares over stoma opening.	
——	——	——	17. Apply skin protectant to a 2″ (5-cm) radius around the stoma, and allow it to dry completely, which takes about 30 seconds.	
——	——	——	18. Lift the gauze squares for a moment and measure the stoma opening, using the measurement guide. Replace the gauze. Trace the same size opening on the back center of the appliance. Cut the opening 1/8″ larger than the stoma size. Check that the spout is closed and the end cap is in place.	
——	——	——	19. Remove the backing from the appliance. Quickly remove the gauze squares and discard appropriately; ease the appliance over the stoma. *Gently press onto the skin while smoothing over the surface. Apply gentle pressure to appliance for a few minutes.*	
——	——	——	20. Secure optional belt to appliance and around patient.	
——	——	——	21. Remove gloves. Assist the patient to a comfortable position. Cover the patient with bed linens. Place the bed in the lowest position.	
——	——	——	22. Put on clean gloves. Remove or discard any remaining equipment and assess patient's response to procedure.	
——	——	——	23. Remove gloves and additional PPE, if used. Perform hand hygiene.	

Skill Checklists for Fundamentals of Nursing:
The Art and Science of Nursing Care, 7th edition

Name _____ Date _____

Unit _____ Position _____

Instructor/Evaluator: _____ Position _____

			SKILL 37-10	
			Caring for a Hemodialysis Access (Arteriovenous Fistula or Graft)	

Goal: The graft or fistula remains patent; the patient verbalizes appropriate care measures and observations to be made, and demonstrates care measures.

Excellent	Satisfactory	Needs Practice		Comments
___	___	___	1. Perform hand hygiene and put on PPE, if indicated.	
___	___	___	2. Identify the patient.	
___	___	___	3. Close curtains around bed and close door to room if possible. Explain what you are going to do, and why you are going to do it, to the patient.	
___	___	___	4. *Inspect area over access site for any redness, warmth, tenderness, or blemishes. Palpate over access site, feeling for a thrill or vibration. Palpate pulses distal to the site. Auscultate over access site with bell of stethoscope, listening for a bruit or vibration.*	
___	___	___	5. Ensure that a sign is placed over head of bed informing the healthcare team which arm is affected. *Do not measure blood pressure, perform a venipuncture, or start an IV on the access arm.*	
___	___	___	6. Instruct patient not to sleep with the arm with the access site under head or body.	
___	___	___	7. Instruct patient not to lift heavy objects with, or put pressure on, the arm with the access site. Advise the patient not to carry heavy bags (including purses) on the shoulder of that arm.	
___	___	___	8. Remove PPE, if used. Perform hand hygiene.	

Skill Checklists for Fundamentals of Nursing:
The Art and Science of Nursing Care, 7th edition

Name _____   Date _____

Unit _____   Position _____

Instructor/Evaluator: _____   Position _____

Excellent	Satisfactory	Needs Practice	SKILL 37-11 **Caring for a Peritoneal Dialysis Catheter**	Comments
			Goal: The peritoneal dialysis catheter dressing change is completed using aseptic technique without trauma to the site or patient; the site is clean, dry, and intact, without evidence of inflammation or infection.	
___	___	___	1. Bring necessary equipment to the bedside stand or overbed table.	
___	___	___	2. Perform hand hygiene and put on PPE, if indicated.	
___	___	___	3. Identify the patient.	
___	___	___	4. Close curtains around bed and close door to room if possible. Explain what you are going to do and why you are going to do it to the patient. Encourage patient to observe or participate if possible.	
___	___	___	5. Adjust bed to comfortable working height, usually elbow height of the caregiver (VISN 8, 2009). Assist patient to a supine position. Expose the abdomen, draping the patient's chest with the bath blanket, exposing only the catheter site.	
___	___	___	6. Put on unsterile gloves. Put on one of the face masks; have patient put on the other mask.	
___	___	___	7. Gently remove old dressing, noting odor, amount, and color of drainage; leakage; and condition of skin around catheter. Discard dressing in appropriate container.	
___	___	___	8. Remove gloves and discard. Set up sterile field. Open packages. Using aseptic technique, place two sterile gauze squares in basin with antimicrobial agent. Leave two sterile gauze squares opened on sterile field. Alternately (based on facility's policy), place sterile antimicrobial swabs on the sterile field. Place sterile applicator on field. Squeeze a small amount of the topical antibiotic on one of the gauze squares on the sterile field.	
___	___	___	9. Put on sterile gloves. Pick up dialysis catheter with nondominant hand. *With the antimicrobial-soaked gauze or swab, cleanse the skin around the exit site using a circular motion, starting at the exit site and then slowly going outward 3" to 4". Gently remove crusted scabs if necessary.*	
___	___	___	10. *Continue to hold catheter with nondominant hand. After skin has dried, clean the catheter with an antimicrobial-soaked gauze, beginning at exit site, going around catheter, and then moving up to end of catheter. Gently remove crusted secretions on the tube if necessary.*	

SKILL 37-11

Caring for a Peritoneal Dialysis Catheter *(Continued)*

Excellent	Satisfactory	Needs Practice		Comments
——	——	——	11. Using the sterile applicator, apply the topical antibiotic to the catheter exit site, if prescribed.	
——	——	——	12. Place sterile drain sponge around exit site. Then place a 4 × 4 gauze over exit site. Remove your gloves and secure edges of gauze pad with tape. Some institutions recommend placing a transparent dressing over the gauze pads instead of tape. Remove masks.	
——	——	——	13. Coil the exposed length of tubing and secure to the dressing or patient's abdomen with tape.	
——	——	——	14. Assist the patient to a comfortable position. Cover the patient with bed linens. Place the bed in the lowest position.	
——	——	——	15. Put on clean gloves. Remove or discard equipment and assess patient's response to procedure.	
——	——	——	16. Remove gloves and additional PPE, if used. Perform hand hygiene.	

Skill Checklists for Fundamentals of Nursing:
The Art and Science of Nursing Care, 7th edition

Name _____ Date _____

Unit _____ Position _____

Instructor/Evaluator: _____ Position _____

SKILL 38-1

Administering a Large-Volume Cleansing Enema

Goal: The patient expels feces and is free from injury with minimal discomfort.

Excellent	Satisfactory	Needs Practice		Comments
——	——	——	1. Verify the order for the enema. Bring necessary equipment to the bedside stand or overbed table.	
——	——	——	2. Perform hand hygiene and put on PPE, if indicated.	
——	——	——	3. Identify the patient.	
——	——	——	4. Close curtains around the bed and close door to room if possible. Explain what you are going to do and why you are going to do it to the patient. Discuss where the patient will defecate. Have a bedpan, commode, or nearby bathroom ready for use.	
——	——	——	5. Warm solution in amount ordered, and check temperature with a bath thermometer if available. If bath thermometer is not available, warm to room temperature or slightly higher, and test on inner wrist. If tap water is used, adjust temperature as it flows from faucet.	
——	——	——	6. Add enema solution to container. Release clamp and allow fluid to progress through tube before reclamping.	
——	——	——	7. Adjust bed to comfortable working height, usually elbow height of the caregiver (VISN 8, 2009). Position the patient on the left side (Sims' position), as dictated by patient comfort and condition. Fold top linen back just enough to allow access to the patient's rectal area. Place a waterproof pad under the patient's hip.	
——	——	——	8. Put on nonsterile gloves.	
——	——	——	9. Elevate solution so that it is no higher than 18″ (45 cm) above level of anus. Plan to give the solution slowly over a period of 5 to 10 minutes. Hang the container on an IV pole or hold it at the proper height.	
——	——	——	10. Generously lubricate end of rectal tube 2″ to 3″ (5–7 cm). A disposable enema set may have a prelubricated rectal tube.	
——	——	——	11. Lift buttock to expose anus. Slowly and gently insert the enema tube 3″ to 4″ (7–10 cm) for an adult. Direct it at an angle pointing toward the umbilicus, not bladder. Ask patient to take several deep breaths.	

Excellent	Satisfactory	Needs Practice	SKILL 38-1 **Administering a Large-Volume Cleansing Enema** *(Continued)*	
				Comments
——	——	——	12. If resistance is met while inserting tube, permit a small amount of solution to enter, withdraw tube slightly, and then continue to insert it. ***Do not force entry of the tube.*** Ask patient to take several deep breaths.	
——	——	——	13. Introduce solution slowly over a period of 5 to 10 minutes. Hold tubing all the time that solution is being instilled.	
——	——	——	14. Clamp tubing or lower container if patient has desire to defecate or cramping occurs. Instruct the patient to take small, fast breaths or to pant.	
——	——	——	15. After solution has been given, clamp tubing and remove tube. Have paper towel ready to receive tube as it is withdrawn.	
——	——	——	16. Return the patient to a comfortable position. Encourage the patient to hold the solution until the urge to defecate is strong, usually in about 5 to 15 minutes. Make sure the linens under the patient are dry. Remove your gloves and ensure that the patient is covered.	
——	——	——	17. Raise side rail. Lower bed height and adjust head of bed to a comfortable position.	
——	——	——	18. Remove additional PPE, if used. Perform hand hygiene.	
——	——	——	19. When patient has a strong urge to defecate, place him or her in a sitting position on a bedpan or assist to commode or bathroom. Offer toilet tissue, if not in patient's reach. Stay with patient or have call bell readily accessible.	
——	——	——	20. Remind patient not to flush commode before nurse inspects results of enema.	
——	——	——	21. Put on gloves and assist patient if necessary with cleaning of anal area. Offer washcloths, soap, and water for hand-washing. Remove gloves.	
——	——	——	22. Leave the patient clean and comfortable. Care for equipment properly.	
——	——	——	23. Perform hand hygiene.	

Skill Checklists for Fundamentals of Nursing:
The Art and Science of Nursing Care, 7th edition

Name _____ Date _____

Unit _____ Position _____

Instructor/Evaluator: _____ Position _____

Excellent	Satisfactory	Needs Practice	SKILL 38-2 **Irrigating a Nasogastric Tube Connected to Suction** **Goal:** The tube maintains patency with irrigation and patient remains free from injury.	Comments
⎯⎯	⎯⎯	⎯⎯	1. Assemble equipment. Verify the medical order or facility policy and procedure regarding frequency of irrigation, solution type, and amount of irrigant. Check expiration dates on irrigating solution and irrigation set.	
⎯⎯	⎯⎯	⎯⎯	2. Perform hand hygiene and put on PPE, if indicated.	
⎯⎯	⎯⎯	⎯⎯	3. Identify the patient.	
⎯⎯	⎯⎯	⎯⎯	4. Explain the procedure to the patient and why this intervention is needed. Answer any questions as needed. Perform key abdominal assessments as described above.	
⎯⎯	⎯⎯	⎯⎯	5. Pull the patient's bedside curtain. Raise bed to a comfortable working position, usually elbow height of the caregiver (VISN 8, 2009). Assist patient to 30- to 45-degree position, unless this is contraindicated. Pour the irrigating solution into container.	
⎯⎯	⎯⎯	⎯⎯	6. Put on gloves. *Check placement of NG tube.*	
⎯⎯	⎯⎯	⎯⎯	7. Draw up 30 mL of saline solution (or amount indicated in the order or policy) into syringe.	
⎯⎯	⎯⎯	⎯⎯	8. Clamp suction tubing near connection site. If needed, disconnect tube from suction apparatus and lay on disposable pad or towel, or hold both tubes upright in nondominant hand.	
⎯⎯	⎯⎯	⎯⎯	9. Place tip of syringe in tube. *If Salem sump or double-lumen tube is used, make sure that the syringe tip is placed in drainage port and not in blue air vent.* Hold syringe upright and gently insert the irrigant (or allow solution to flow in by gravity if agency policy or physician indicates). *Do not force solution into tube.*	
⎯⎯	⎯⎯	⎯⎯	10. *If unable to irrigate tube, reposition patient and attempt irrigation again. Inject 10 to 20 mL of air and aspirate again. Check with physician or follow agency policy if repeated attempts to irrigate tube fail.*	

Excellent	Satisfactory	Needs Practice		Comments
——	——	——	11. After irrigant has been instilled, hold end of NG tube over irrigation tray or emesis basin. Observe for return flow of NG drainage into available container. Alternately, the nurse may reconnect the NG tube to suction and observe the return drainage as it drains into the suction container.	
——	——	——	12. *If not already done, reconnect drainage port to suction, if ordered.*	
——	——	——	13. *Inject air into blue air vent after irrigation is complete. Position the blue air vent above the patient's stomach.*	
——	——	——	14. Remove gloves. Lower the bed and raise side rails, as necessary. Assist the patient to a position of comfort. Perform hand hygiene.	
——	——	——	15. Put on gloves. Measure returned solution, if collected outside of suction apparatus. Rinse equipment if it will be reused. Label with the date, patient's name, room number, and purpose (for NG tube/ irrigation).	
——	——	——	16. Remove gloves and additional PPE, if used. Perform hand hygiene.	

Skill Checklists for Fundamentals of Nursing:
The Art and Science of Nursing Care, 7th edition

Name _____   Date _____

Unit _____   Position _____

Instructor/Evaluator: _____   Position _____

Excellent	Satisfactory	Needs Practice	SKILL 38-3 **Changing and Emptying an Ostomy Appliance**	Comments
			Goal: The stoma appliance is applied correctly to the skin to allow stool to drain freely.	
——	——	——	1. Bring necessary equipment to the bedside stand or overbed table.	
——	——	——	2. Perform hand hygiene and put on PPE, if indicated.	
——	——	——	3. Identify the patient.	
——	——	——	4. Close curtains around bed and close door to room if possible. Explain what you are going to do and why you are going to do it to the patient. Encourage patient to observe or participate if possible.	
——	——	——	5. Assist patient to a comfortable sitting or lying position in bed or a standing or sitting position in the bathroom.	
			Emptying an Appliance	
——	——	——	6. Put on disposable gloves. Remove clamp and fold end of pouch upward like a cuff.	
——	——	——	7. Empty contents into bedpan, toilet, or measuring device.	
——	——	——	8. Wipe the lower 2″ of the appliance or pouch with toilet tissue.	
——	——	——	9. Uncuff edge of appliance or pouch and apply clip or clamp, or secure Velcro closure. Ensure the curve of the clamp follows the curve of the patient's body. Remove gloves. Assist patient to a comfortable position.	
——	——	——	10. If appliance is not to be changed, remove additional PPE, if used. Perform hand hygiene.	
			Changing an Appliance	
——	——	——	11. Place a disposable pad on the work surface. Set up the washbasin with warm water and the rest of the supplies. Place a trash bag within reach.	
——	——	——	12. Put on clean gloves. Place waterproof pad under the patient at the stoma site. Empty the appliance, as described previously.	

Excellent	Satisfactory	Needs Practice	SKILL 38-3
			Changing and Emptying an Ostomy Appliance

Comments

——	——	——	13. Gently remove pouch faceplate from skin by pushing skin from appliance rather than pulling appliance from skin. Start at the top of the appliance, while keeping the abdominal skin taut. Apply a silicone-based adhesive remover by spraying or wiping with the remover wipe.
——	——	——	14. Place the appliance in the trash bag, if disposable. If reusable, set aside to wash in lukewarm soap and water and allow to air dry after the new appliance is in place.
——	——	——	15. Use toilet tissue to remove any excess stool from stoma. Cover stoma with gauze pad. Clean skin around stoma with mild soap and water or a cleansing agent and a washcloth. Remove all old adhesive from skin; use an adhesive remover as necessary. Do not apply lotion to peristomal area.
——	——	——	16. Gently pat area dry. Make sure skin around stoma is thoroughly dry. Assess stoma and condition of surrounding skin.
——	——	——	17. Apply skin protectant to a 2″ (5-cm) radius around the stoma, and allow it to dry completely, which takes about 30 seconds.
——	——	——	18. Lift the gauze squares for a moment and measure the stoma opening, using the measurement guide. Replace the gauze. Trace the same-size opening on the back center of the appliance. Cut the opening 1/8″ larger than the stoma size.
——	——	——	19. Remove the backing from the appliance. Quickly remove the gauze squares and ease the appliance over the stoma. Gently press onto the skin while smoothing over the surface. Apply gentle pressure to appliance for 5 minutes.
——	——	——	20. Close bottom of appliance or pouch by folding the end upward and using clamp or clip that comes with product, or secure Velcro closure. Ensure the curve of the clamp follows the curve of the patient's body.
——	——	——	21. Remove gloves. Assist the patient to a comfortable position. Cover the patient with bed linens. Place the bed in the lowest position.
——	——	——	22. Put on clean gloves. Remove or discard equipment and assess patient's response to procedure.
——	——	——	23. Remove gloves and additional PPE, if used. Perform hand hygiene.

Skill Checklists for Fundamentals of Nursing:
The Art and Science of Nursing Care, 7th edition

Name _____   Date _____

Unit _____   Position _____

Instructor/Evaluator: _____   Position _____

Excellent	Satisfactory	Needs Practice	SKILL 39-1 **Using a Pulse Oximeter**	Comments
			Goal: The patient exhibits arterial blood oxygen saturation within acceptable parameters, or greater than 95%.	
——	——	——	1. Review chart for any health problems that would affect the patient's oxygenation status.	
——	——	——	2. Bring necessary equipment to the bedside stand or overbed table.	
——	——	——	3. Perform hand hygiene and put on PPE, if indicated.	
——	——	——	4. Identify the patient.	
——	——	——	5. Close curtains around bed and close door to room if possible. Explain what you are going to do and why you are going to do it to the patient.	
——	——	——	6. Select an adequate site for application of the sensor.	
——	——	——	a. Use the patient's index, middle, or ring finger.	
——	——	——	b. Check the proximal pulse and capillary refill at the pulse closest to the site.	
——	——	——	c. If circulation at site is inadequate, consider using the earlobe, forehead, or bridge of nose.	
——	——	——	d. Use a toe only if lower extremity circulation is not compromised.	
——	——	——	7. Select proper equipment:	
——	——	——	a. If one finger is too large for the probe, use a smaller one. A pediatric probe may be used for a small adult.	
——	——	——	b. Use probes appropriate for patient's age and size.	
——	——	——	c. Check if patient is allergic to adhesive. A nonadhesive finger clip or reflectance sensor is available.	
——	——	——	8. Prepare the monitoring site. Cleanse the selected area with the alcohol wipe or disposable cleansing cloth. Allow the area to dry. If necessary, remove nail polish and artificial nails after checking pulse oximeter's manufacturer instructions.	
——	——	——	9. *Apply probe securely to skin. Make sure that the light-emitting sensor and the light-receiving sensor are aligned opposite each other (not necessary to check if placed on forehead or bridge of nose).*	

Excellent	Satisfactory	Needs Practice	SKILL 39-1 **Using a Pulse Oximeter** *(Continued)*	Comments
⎯	⎯	⎯	10. Connect the sensor probe to the pulse oximeter, turn the oximeter on, and check operation of the equipment (audible beep, fluctuation of bar of light or waveform on face of oximeter).	
⎯	⎯	⎯	11. Set alarms on pulse oximeter. Check manufacturer's alarm limits for high and low pulse rate settings.	
⎯	⎯	⎯	12. Check oxygen saturation at regular intervals, as ordered by primary care provider, nursing assessment, and signaled by alarms. Monitor hemoglobin level.	
⎯	⎯	⎯	13. Remove sensor on a regular basis and check for skin irritation or signs of pressure (every 2 hours for spring tension sensor or every 4 hours for adhesive finger or toe sensor).	
⎯	⎯	⎯	14. Clean nondisposable sensors according to the manufacturer's directions. Remove PPE, if used. Perform hand hygiene.	

Skill Checklists for Fundamentals of Nursing:
The Art and Science of Nursing Care, 7th edition

Name _____ Date _____

Unit _____ Position _____

Instructor/Evaluator: _____ Position _____

SKILL 39-2

Suctioning the Nasopharyngeal and Oropharyngeal Airways

Goal: The patient exhibits improved breath sounds and a clear, patent airway.

Excellent	Satisfactory	Needs Practice		Comments
—	—	—	1. Bring necessary equipment to the bedside stand or overbed table.	
—	—	—	2. Perform hand hygiene and put on PPE, if indicated.	
—	—	—	3. Identify the patient.	
—	—	—	4. Close curtains around bed and close door to room if possible.	
—	—	—	5. Determine the need for suctioning. Verify the suction order in the patient's chart, if necessary. *For postoperative patient, administer pain medication before suctioning.*	
—	—	—	6. Explain what you are going to do and the reason for suctioning to the patient, even if the patient does not appear to be alert. Reassure patient you will interrupt procedure if he or she indicates respiratory difficulty.	
—	—	—	7. Adjust bed to comfortable working height, usually elbow height of the caregiver (VISN 8, 2009). Lower side rail closest to you. *If patient is conscious, place him or her in a semi-Fowler's position. If patient is unconscious, place him or her in the lateral position, facing you.* Move the bed table close to your work area and raise to waist height.	
—	—	—	8. Place towel or waterproof pad across the patient's chest.	
—	—	—	9. *Adjust suction to appropriate pressure.*	
—	—	—	For a wall unit for an adult: 100–120 mm Hg (Roman, 2005); neonates: 60–80 mm Hg; infants: 80–100 mm Hg; children: 80–100 mm Hg; adolescents: 80–120 mm Hg (Ireton, 2007).	
—	—	—	For a portable unit for an adult: 10–15 cm Hg; neonates: 6–8 cm Hg; infants: 8–10 cm Hg; children: 8–10 cm Hg; adolescents: 8–10 cm Hg.	
—	—	—	*Put on a disposable, clean glove and occlude the end of the connecting tubing to check suction pressure.* Place the connecting tubing in a convenient location.	

Excellent	Satisfactory	Needs Practice	SKILL 39-2 **Suctioning the Nasopharyngeal and Oropharyngeal Airways** *(Continued)*	Comments
——	——	——	10. Open sterile suction package using aseptic technique. The open wrapper or container becomes a sterile field to hold other supplies. Carefully remove the sterile container, touching only the outside surface. Set it up on the work surface and pour sterile saline into it.	
——	——	——	11. Place a small amount of water-soluble lubricant on the sterile field, taking care to avoid touching the sterile field with the lubricant package.	
——	——	——	12. Increase the patient's supplemental oxygen level or apply supplemental oxygen per facility policy or primary care provider order.	
——	——	——	13. Put on face shield or goggles and mask. Put on sterile gloves. *The dominant hand will manipulate the catheter and must remain sterile. The nondominant hand is considered clean rather than sterile and will control the suction valve (Y port) on the catheter.*	
——	——	——	14. With dominant gloved hand, pick up sterile catheter. Pick up the connecting tubing with the nondominant hand and connect the tubing and suction catheter.	
——	——	——	15. Moisten the catheter by dipping it into the container of sterile saline. Occlude Y-tube to check suction.	
——	——	——	16. Encourage the patient to take several deep breaths.	
——	——	——	17. Apply lubricant to the first 2″ to 3″ of the catheter, using the lubricant that was placed on the sterile field.	
——	——	——	18. Remove the oxygen delivery device, if appropriate. Do not apply suction as the catheter is inserted. Hold the catheter between your thumb and forefinger.	
——	——	——	19. Insert the catheter:	
——	——	——	a. For nasopharyngeal suctioning, gently insert catheter through the naris and along the floor of the nostril toward the trachea. Roll the catheter between your fingers to help advance it. Advance the catheter approximately 5″ to 6″ to reach the pharynx.	
——	——	——	b. For oropharyngeal suctioning, insert catheter through the mouth, along the side of the mouth toward the trachea. Advance the catheter 3″ to 4″ to reach the pharynx.	
——	——	——	20. Apply suction by intermittently occluding the Y port on the catheter with the thumb of your nondominant hand and gently rotate the catheter as it is being withdrawn. *Do not suction for more than 10 to 15 seconds at a time.*	

Suctioning the Nasopharyngeal and Oropharyngeal Airways *(Continued)*

Excellent	Satisfactory	Needs Practice		Comments
——	——	——	21. Replace the oxygen-delivery device using your nondominant hand, if appropriate, and have the patient take several deep breaths.	
——	——	——	22. Flush catheter with saline. Assess effectiveness of suctioning and repeat as needed and according to patient's tolerance. Wrap the suction catheter around your dominant hand between attempts.	
——	——	——	23. *Allow at least a 30-second to 1-minute interval if additional suctioning is needed. No more than three suction passes should be made per suctioning episode. Alternate the nares, unless contraindicated, if repeated suctioning is required.* Do not force catheter through the nares. Encourage patient to cough and deep breathe between suctioning. Suction the oropharynx after suctioning the nasopharynx.	
——	——	——	24. When suctioning is completed, remove gloves from dominant hand over the coiled catheter, pulling it off inside out. Remove glove from nondominant hand and dispose of gloves, catheter, and container with solution in the appropriate receptacle. Assist patient to a comfortable position. Raise bed rail and place bed in the lowest position.	
——	——	——	25. Turn off suction. Remove supplemental oxygen placed for suctioning, if appropriate. Remove face shield or goggles and mask. Perform hand hygiene.	
——	——	——	26. Offer oral hygiene after suctioning.	
——	——	——	27. Reassess patient's respiratory status, including respiratory rate, effort, oxygen saturation, and lung sounds.	
——	——	——	28. Remove additional PPE, if used. Perform hand hygiene.	

Skill Checklists for Fundamentals of Nursing:
The Art and Science of Nursing Care, 7th edition

Name _____ Date _____

Unit _____ Position _____

Instructor/Evaluator: _____ Position _____

SKILL 39-3

Administering Oxygen by Nasal Cannula

Excellent	Satisfactory	Needs Practice	**Goal:** The patient exhibits an oxygen saturation level within acceptable parameters.	Comments
——	——	——	1. Bring necessary equipment to the bedside stand or overbed table.	
——	——	——	2. Perform hand hygiene and put on PPE, if indicated.	
——	——	——	3. Identify the patient.	
——	——	——	4. Close curtains around bed and close door to room if possible.	
——	——	——	5. Explain what you are going to do and the reason for doing it to the patient. Review safety precautions necessary when oxygen is in use. Place "No Smoking" signs in appropriate areas.	
——	——	——	6. Connect nasal cannula to oxygen setup with humidification, if one is in use. Adjust flow rate as ordered. Check that oxygen is flowing out of prongs.	
——	——	——	7. Place prongs in patient's nostrils. Place tubing over and behind each ear with adjuster comfortably under chin. Alternately, the tubing may be placed around the patient's head, with adjuster at the back or base of the head. Place gauze pads at ear beneath the tubing as necessary.	
——	——	——	8. Adjust the fit of the cannula as necessary. Tubing should be snug but not tight against the skin.	
——	——	——	9. *Encourage patients to breathe through the nose, with the mouth closed.*	
——	——	——	10. Reassess patient's respiratory status, including respiratory rate, effort, and lung sounds. Note any signs of respiratory distress, such as tachypnea, nasal flaring, use of accessory muscles, or dyspnea.	
——	——	——	11. Remove PPE, if used. Perform hand hygiene.	
——	——	——	12. Put on clean gloves. Remove and clean the cannula and assess nares at least every 8 hours, or according to agency recommendations. Check nares for evidence of irritation or bleeding.	

Skill Checklists for Fundamentals of Nursing:
The Art and Science of Nursing Care, 7th edition

Name _____ Date _____

Unit _____ Position _____

Instructor/Evaluator: _____ Position _____

Excellent	Satisfactory	Needs Practice	SKILL 39-4 **Administering Oxygen by Mask**	Comments
			Goal: The patient exhibits an oxygen saturation level within acceptable parameters.	
——	——	——	1. Bring necessary equipment to the bedside stand or overbed table.	
——	——	——	2. Perform hand hygiene and put on PPE, if indicated.	
——	——	——	3. Identify the patient.	
——	——	——	4. Close curtains around bed and close door to room if possible.	
——	——	——	5. Explain what you are going to do and the reason for doing it to the patient. Review safety precautions necessary when oxygen is in use. Place "No Smoking" signs in appropriate areas.	
——	——	——	6. Attach face mask to oxygen source (with humidification, if appropriate, for the specific mask). Start the flow of oxygen at the specified rate. For a mask with a reservoir, be sure to allow oxygen to fill the bag before proceeding to the next step.	
——	——	——	7. Position face mask over patient's nose and mouth. Adjust the elastic strap so that the mask fits snugly but comfortably on the face. Adjust the flow rate to the prescribed rate.	
——	——	——	8. If the patient reports irritation or redness is noted, use gauze pads under the elastic strap at pressure points to reduce irritation to ears and scalp.	
——	——	——	9. Reassess patient's respiratory status, including respiratory rate, effort, and lung sounds. Note any signs of respiratory distress, such as tachypnea, nasal flaring, use of accessory muscles, or dyspnea.	
——	——	——	10. Remove PPE, if used. Perform hand hygiene.	
——	——	——	11. *Remove the mask and dry the skin every 2 to 3 hours if the oxygen is running continuously. Do not use powder around the mask.*	

Skill Checklists for Fundamentals of Nursing:
The Art and Science of Nursing Care, 7th edition

Name _____ Date _____

Unit _____ Position _____

Instructor/Evaluator: _____ Position _____

Excellent	Satisfactory	Needs Practice	SKILL 39-5 **Suctioning the Tracheostomy: Open System**	
			Goal: The patient exhibits improved breath sounds and a clear, patent airway.	**Comments**
——	——	——	1. Bring necessary equipment to the bedside stand or overbed table.	
——	——	——	2. Perform hand hygiene and put on PPE, if indicated.	
——	——	——	3. Identify the patient.	
——	——	——	4. Close curtains around bed and close door to room if possible.	
——	——	——	5. Determine the need for suctioning. Verify the suction order in the patient's chart. *Assess for pain or the potential to cause pain. Administer pain medication as prescribed before suctioning.*	
——	——	——	6. Explain to the patient what you are going to do and the reason for doing it, even if the patient does not appear to be alert. Reassure patient you will interrupt procedure if he or she indicates respiratory difficulty.	
——	——	——	7. Adjust bed to comfortable working position, usually elbow height of the caregiver (VISN 8, 2009). Lower side rail closest to you. *If patient is conscious, place him or her in a semi-Fowler's position. If patient is unconscious, place him or her in the lateral position, facing you.* Move the overbed table close to your work area and raise to waist height.	
——	——	——	8. Place towel or waterproof pad across patient's chest.	
——	——	——	9. *Turn suction to appropriate pressure.*	
——	——	——	For a wall unit for an adult: 100–120 mm Hg (Roman, 2005); neonates: 60–80 mm Hg; infants: 80–100 mm Hg; children: 80–100 mm Hg; adolescents: 80–120 mm Hg (Ireton, 2007).	
——	——	——	For a portable unit for an adult: 10–15 cm Hg; neonates: 6–8 cm Hg; infants: 8–10 cm Hg; children: 8–10 cm Hg; adolescents: 8–10 cm Hg.	
——	——	——	*Put on a disposable, clean glove and occlude the end of the connecting tubing to check suction pressure. Place the connecting tubing in a convenient location. If using, place resuscitation bag connected to oxygen within convenient reach.*	

Suctioning the Tracheostomy: Open System *(Continued)*

Excellent	Satisfactory	Needs Practice		Comments

Comments

10. Open sterile suction package using aseptic technique. The open wrapper or container becomes a sterile field to hold other supplies. Carefully remove the sterile container, touching only the outside surface. Set it up on the work surface and pour sterile saline into it.

11. Put on face shield or goggles and mask. Put on sterile gloves. *The dominant hand will manipulate the catheter and must remain sterile. The nondominant hand is considered clean rather than sterile and will control the suction valve (Y port) on the catheter.*

12. With dominant gloved hand, pick up sterile catheter. Pick up the connecting tubing with the nondominant hand and connect the tubing and suction catheter.

13. Moisten the catheter by dipping it into the container of sterile saline, unless it is a silicone catheter. Occlude Y-tube to check suction.

14. Using your nondominant hand and a manual resuscitation bag, hyperventilate the patient, delivering 3 to 6 breaths or use the sigh mechanism on a mechanical ventilator.

15. Open the adapter on the mechanical ventilator tubing or remove oxygen delivery setup with your nondominant hand.

16. Using your dominant hand, gently and quickly insert catheter into trachea. *Advance the catheter to the predetermined length. Do not occlude Y-port when inserting catheter.*

17. Apply suction by intermittently occluding the Y port on the catheter with the thumb of your nondominant hand, and gently rotate the catheter as it is being withdrawn. *Do not suction for more than 10 to 15 seconds at a time.*

18. Hyperventilate the patient using your nondominant hand and a manual resuscitation bag, delivering 3 to 6 breaths. Replace the oxygen delivery device, if applicable, using your nondominant hand and have the patient take several deep breaths. If the patient is mechanically ventilated, close the adapter on the mechanical ventilator tubing and use the sigh mechanism on a mechanical ventilator.

19. Flush catheter with saline. Assess effectiveness of suctioning and repeat as needed and according to patient's tolerance. Wrap the suction catheter around your dominant hand between attempts.

Excellent	Satisfactory	Needs Practice		Comments
			SKILL 39-5 **Suctioning the Tracheostomy: Open System** *(Continued)*	
——	——	——	20. *Allow at least a 30-second to 1-minute interval if additional suctioning is needed. No more than three suction passes should be made per suctioning episode. Encourage patient to cough and deep breathe between suctionings.* Suction the oropharynx after suctioning the trachea. Do not reinsert in the tracheostomy after suctioning the mouth.	
——	——	——	21. When suctioning is completed, remove gloves from dominant hand over the coiled catheter, pulling it off inside out. Remove glove from nondominant hand and dispose of gloves, catheter, and container with solution in the appropriate receptacle. Assist patient to a comfortable position. Raise bed rail and place bed in the lowest position.	
——	——	——	22. Turn off suction. Remove supplemental oxygen placed for suctioning, if appropriate. Remove face shield or goggles and mask. Perform hand hygiene.	
——	——	——	23. Offer oral hygiene after suctioning.	
——	——	——	24. Reassess patient's respiratory status, including respiratory rate, effort, oxygen saturation, and lung sounds.	
——	——	——	25. Remove additional PPE, if used. Perform hand hygiene.	

Skill Checklists for Fundamentals of Nursing:
The Art and Science of Nursing Care, 7th edition

Name _____ Date _____

Unit _____ Position _____

Instructor/Evaluator: _____ Position _____

SKILL 39-6

Providing Tracheostomy Care

Goal: The patient exhibits a tracheostomy tube and site free from drainage, secretions, and skin irritation or breakdown.

Excellent	Satisfactory	Needs Practice		Comments
――	――	――	1. Bring necessary equipment to the bedside stand or overbed table.	
――	――	――	2. Perform hand hygiene and put on PPE, if indicated.	
――	――	――	3. Identify the patient.	
――	――	――	4. Close curtains around bed and close door to room if possible.	
――	――	――	5. Determine the need for tracheostomy care. *Assess patient's pain and administer pain medication, if indicated.*	
――	――	――	6. Explain what you are going to do and the reason to the patient, even if the patient does not appear to be alert. Reassure patient you will interrupt procedure if he or she indicates respiratory difficulty.	
――	――	――	7. Adjust bed to comfortable working position, usually elbow height of the caregiver (VISN 8, 2009). Lower side rail closest to you. *If patient is conscious, place him or her in a semi-Fowler's position. If patient is unconscious, place him or her in the lateral position, facing you.* Move the overbed table close to your work area and raise to waist height. Place a trash receptacle within easy reach of work area.	
――	――	――	8. Put on face shield or goggles and mask. Suction tracheostomy if necessary. If tracheostomy has just been suctioned, remove soiled site dressing and discard before removal of gloves used to perform suctioning.	

Cleaning the Tracheostomy: Disposable Inner Cannula

Excellent	Satisfactory	Needs Practice		Comments
――	――	――	9. Carefully open the package with the new disposable inner cannula, taking care not to contaminate the cannula or the inside of the package. Carefully open the package with the sterile cotton-tipped applicators, taking care not to contaminate them. Open sterile cup or basin and fill 0.5 inches deep with saline. Open the plastic disposable bag and place within reach on work surface.	
――	――	――	10. Put on disposable gloves.	

SKILL 39-6

Providing Tracheostomy Care (Continued)

Excellent	Satisfactory	Needs Practice		Comments
——	——	——	11. Remove the oxygen source if one is present. Stabilize the outer cannula and faceplate of the tracheostomy with your nondominant hand. Grasp the locking mechanism of the inner cannula with your dominant hand. Press the tabs and release lock. Gently remove inner cannula and place in disposal bag. If not already removed, remove site dressing and dispose of in the trash.	
——	——	——	12. Discard gloves and put on sterile gloves. Pick up the new inner cannula with your dominant hand, stabilize the faceplate with your nondominant hand, and gently insert the new inner cannula into the outer cannula. Press the tabs to allow the lock to grab the outer cannula. Reapply oxygen source if needed.	

Applying Clean Dressing and Holder

Excellent	Satisfactory	Needs Practice		Comments
——	——	——	13. Remove oxygen source, if necessary. Dip cotton-tipped applicator or gauze sponge in cup or basin with sterile saline and clean stoma under faceplate. *Use each applicator or sponge only once, moving from stoma site outward.*	
——	——	——	14. Pat skin gently with dry 4″ × 4″ gauze sponge.	
——	——	——	15. Slide commercially prepared tracheostomy dressing or pre-folded noncotton-filled 4″ × 4″ dressing under the faceplate.	
——	——	——	16. Change the tracheostomy holder:	
——	——	——	a. *Obtain the assistance of a second individual to hold the tracheostomy tube in place while the old collar is removed and the new collar is placed.*	
——	——	——	b. Open the package for the new tracheostomy collar.	
——	——	——	c. Both nurses should put on clean gloves.	
——	——	——	d. One nurse holds the faceplate while the other pulls up the Velcro tabs. Gently remove the collar.	
——	——	——	e. The first nurse continues to hold the tracheostomy faceplate.	
——	——	——	f. The other nurse places the collar around the patient's neck and inserts first one tab, then the other, into the openings on the faceplate and secures the Velcro tabs on the tracheostomy holder.	
——	——	——	g. Check the fit of the tracheostomy collar. You should be able to fit one finger between the neck and the collar. Check to make sure that the patient can flex neck comfortably. Reapply oxygen source if necessary.	

SKILL 39-6

Providing Tracheostomy Care *(Continued)*

Excellent	Satisfactory	Needs Practice		Comments
——	——	——	17. Remove gloves. Assist patient to a comfortable position. Raise the bed rail and place the bed in the lowest position.	
——	——	——	18. Remove face shield or goggles and mask. Remove additional PPE, if used. Perform hand hygiene.	
——	——	——	19. Reassess patient's respiratory status, including respiratory rate, effort, oxygen saturation, and lung sounds.	

Skill Checklists for Fundamentals of Nursing:
The Art and Science of Nursing Care, 7th edition

Name _____   Date _____

Unit _____   Position _____

Instructor/Evaluator: _____   Position _____

Excellent	Satisfactory	Needs Practice	SKILL 40-1 **Initiating a Peripheral Venous Access IV Infusion**	
			Goal: The access device is inserted on the first attempt, using sterile technique.	**Comments**
___	___	___	1. Verify the IV solution order on the MAR/CMAR with the medical order. Clarify any inconsistencies. Check the patient's chart for allergies. Check for color, leaking, and expiration date. Know techniques for IV insertion, precautions, purpose of the IV administration, and medications if ordered.	
___	___	___	2. Gather all equipment and bring to the bedside.	
___	___	___	3. Perform hand hygiene and put on PPE, if indicated.	
___	___	___	4. Identify the patient.	
___	___	___	5. Close curtains around bed and close door to the room if possible. Explain what you are going to do and why you are going to do it to the patient. Ask the patient about allergies to medications, tape, or skin antiseptics, as appropriate. If considering using a local anesthetic, inquire about allergies for these substances as well.	
___	___	___	6. If using a local anesthetic, explain the rationale and procedure to the patient. Apply the anesthetic to a few potential insertion sites. Allow sufficient time for the anesthetic to take effect.	
			Prepare the IV Solution and Administration Set	
___	___	___	7. Compare the IV container label with the MAR/CMAR. Remove IV bag from outer wrapper, if indicated. Check expiration dates. Scan bar code on container, if necessary. Compare on patient identification band with the MAR/CMAR. Alternately, label the solution container with the patient's name, solution type, additives, date, and time. Complete a time strip for the infusion and apply to IV container.	
___	___	___	8. Maintain aseptic technique when opening sterile packages and IV solution. Remove administration set from package. Apply label to tubing reflecting the day/date for next set change, per facility guidelines.	

Initiating a Peripheral Venous Access
IV Infusion *(Continued)*

Excellent	Satisfactory	Needs Practice		Comments
——	——	——	9. Close the roller clamp or slide clamp on the IV administration set. Invert the IV solution container and remove the cap on the entry site, taking care to not touch the exposed entry site. Remove the cap from the spike on the administration set. Using a twisting and pushing motion, insert the administration set spike into the entry site of the IV container. Alternately, follow the manufacturer's directions for insertion.	
——	——	——	10. Hang the IV container on the IV pole. Squeeze the drip chamber and fill at least halfway.	
——	——	——	11. Open the IV tubing clamp and allow fluid to move through tubing. Follow additional manufacturer's instructions for specific electronic infusion pump, as indicated. ***Allow fluid to flow until all air bubbles have disappeared and the entire length of the tubing is primed (filled) with IV solution.*** Close clamp. Alternately, some brands of tubing may require removal of cap at end of the IV tubing to allow fluid to flow. Maintain its sterility. After fluid has filled the tubing, recap end of tubing.	
——	——	——	12. If an electronic device is to be used, follow manufacturer's instructions for inserting tubing into the device.	

Initiate Peripheral Venous Access

Excellent	Satisfactory	Needs Practice		Comments
——	——	——	13. Place patient in low Fowler's position in bed. Place protective towel or pad under patient's arm.	
——	——	——	14. Provide emotional support as needed.	
——	——	——	15. Open the short extension tubing package. Attach end cap, if not in place. Clean end cap with alcohol wipe. Insert syringe with normal saline into extension tubing. Fill extension tubing with normal saline and apply slide clamp. Remove the syringe and place extension tubing and syringe back on package, within easy reach.	
——	——	——	16. Select and palpate for an appropriate vein. Refer to guidelines in previous Assessment section.	
——	——	——	17. If the site is hairy and agency policy permits, clip a 2″ area around the intended site of entry.	
——	——	——	18. Put on gloves.	
——	——	——	19. Apply a tourniquet 3″ to 4″ above the venipuncture site to obstruct venous blood flow and distend the vein. Direct the ends of the tourniquet away from the site of entry. Make sure the radial pulse is still present.	

Initiating a Peripheral Venous Access
IV Infusion *(Continued)*

Excellent	Satisfactory	Needs Practice		Comments
——	——	——	20. Instruct the patient to hold the arm lower than the heart.	
——	——	——	21. Ask patient to open and close fist. Observe and palpate for a suitable vein. Try the following techniques if a vein cannot be felt:	
——	——	——	a. Massage the patient's arm from proximal to distal end and gently tap over intended vein.	
——	——	——	b. Remove tourniquet and place warm, moist compresses over intended vein for 10 to 15 minutes.	
——	——	——	22. ***Cleanse site with an antiseptic solution such as chlorhexidine or according to facility policy. Press applicator against the skin and apply chlorhexidine using a back and forth friction scrub for at least 30 seconds. Do not wipe or blot. Allow to dry completely.***	
——	——	——	23. Use the nondominant hand, placed about 1″ or 2″ below entry site, to hold the skin taut against the vein. ***Avoid touching the prepared site.*** Ask the patient to remain still while you are performing the venipuncture.	
——	——	——	24. Enter the skin gently, holding the catheter by the hub in your dominant hand, bevel side up, at a 10- to 15-degree angle. Insert the catheter from directly over the vein or from the side of the vein. While following the course of the vein, advance the needle or catheter into the vein. A sensation of "give" can be felt when the needle enters the vein.	
——	——	——	25. When blood returns through the lumen of the needle or the flashback chamber of the catheter, advance either device into the vein until the hub is at the venipuncture site. The exact technique depends on the type of device used.	
——	——	——	26. Release the tourniquet. Quickly remove the protective cap from the extension tubing and attach to the catheter or needle. Stabilize the catheter or needle with your nondominant hand.	
——	——	——	27. Continue to stabilize the catheter or needle and flush gently with the saline, observing the site for infiltration and leaking.	
——	——	——	28. Open the skin protectant wipe. Apply the skin protectant to the site, making sure to cover at minimum the area to be covered with the dressing. Place sterile transparent dressing or catheter securing/stabilization device over venipuncture site. Loop the tubing near the site of entry, and anchor with tape (nonallergenic) close to site.	

Excellent	Satisfactory	Needs Practice		Comments
			SKILL 40-1 **Initiating a Peripheral Venous Access** **IV Infusion** *(Continued)*	
——	——	——	29. Label the IV dressing with the date, time, site, and type and size of catheter or needle used for the infusion.	
——	——	——	30. Using an antimicrobial swab, cleanse access cap on extension tubing. Remove the end cap from the administration set. Insert the end of the administration set into the end cap. Loop the administration set tubing near the site of entry, and anchor with tape (nonallergenic) close to site. Remove gloves.	
——	——	——	31. Open the clamp on the administration set. Set the rate of flow and begin the fluid infusion. Alternately, start the flow of solution by releasing the clamp on the tubing and counting the drops. Adjust until the correct drop rate is achieved. Assess the flow of the solution and function of the infusion device. Inspect the insertion site for signs of infiltration.	
——	——	——	32. Apply an IV securement/stabilization device if not already in place as part of dressing, as indicated, based on facility policy. Explain to patient the purpose of the device and the importance of safeguarding the site when using the extremity.	
——	——	——	33. Remove equipment and return patient to a position of comfort. Lower bed, if not in lowest position.	
——	——	——	34. Remove additional PPE, if used. Perform hand hygiene.	
——	——	——	35. Return to check flow rate and observe IV site for infiltration 30 minutes after starting infusion, and at least hourly thereafter. Ask the patient if he or she is experiencing any pain or discomfort related to the IV infusion.	

Name _____   Date _____

Unit _____   Position _____

Instructor/Evaluator: _____   Position _____

Excellent	Satisfactory	Needs Practice	SKILL 40-2 ## Changing an IV Solution Container and Administration Set **Goal:** The prescribed IV infusion continues without interruption and with infusion complications identified.	Comments
___	___	___	1. Verify IV solution order on MAR/CMAR with the medical order. Clarify any inconsistencies. Check the patient's chart for allergies. Check for color, leaking, and expiration date. Know the purpose of the IV administration and medications if ordered.	
___	___	___	2. Gather all equipment and bring to bedside.	
___	___	___	3. Perform hand hygiene and put on PPE, if indicated.	
___	___	___	4. Identify the patient.	
___	___	___	5. Close curtains around bed and close door to room if possible. Explain what you are going to do and why you are going to do it to the patient. Ask the patient about allergies to medications or tape, as appropriate.	
___	___	___	6. Compare IV container label with the MAR/CMAR. Remove IV bag from outer wrapper, if indicated. Check expiration dates. Scan bar code on container, if necessary. Compare patient identification band with the MAR/CMAR. Alternately, label solution container with the patient's name, solution type, additives, date, and time. Complete a time strip for the infusion and apply to IV container.	
___	___	___	7. Maintain aseptic technique when opening sterile packages and IV solution. Remove administration set from package. Apply label to tubing reflecting the day/date for next set change, per facility guidelines.	
			To Change IV Solution Container	
___	___	___	8. If using an electronic infusion device, pause the device or put on "hold." Close the slide clamp on the administration set closest to the drip chamber. If using gravity infusion, close the roller clamp on the administration set.	
___	___	___	9. Carefully remove the cap on the entry site of the new IV solution container and expose entry site, taking care to not touch the exposed entry site.	
___	___	___	10. Lift empty container off IV pole and invert it. Quickly remove the spike from the old IV container, *being careful not to contaminate it*. Discard old IV container.	

Changing an IV Solution Container and Administration Set (Continued)

Excellent	Satisfactory	Needs Practice		Comments
——	——	——	11. Using a twisting and pushing motion, insert the administration set spike into the entry site of the IV container. Alternately, follow the manufacturer's directions for insertion. Hang the container on the IV pole.	
——	——	——	12. Alternately, hang the new IV fluid container on an open hook on the IV pole. Carefully remove the cap on the entry site of the new IV solution container and expose entry site, taking care to not touch the exposed entry site. Lift empty container off IV pole and invert it. Quickly remove the spike from the old IV container, **being careful not to contaminate it.** Discard old IV container. Using a twisting and pushing motion, insert the administration set spike into the entry port of the new IV container as it hangs on the IV pole.	
——	——	——	13. If using an electronic infusion device, open the slide clamp, check the drip chamber of the administration set, verify the flow rate programmed in the infusion device, and turn the device to "run" or "infuse."	
——	——	——	14. If using gravity infusion, slowly open the roller clamp on the administration set and count the drops. Adjust until the correct drop rate is achieved.	
			To Change IV Solution Container and Administration Set	
——	——	——	15. Prepare the IV solution and administration set. Refer to Skill 40-1, Steps 7–11.	
——	——	——	16. Hang the IV container on an open hook on the IV pole. Close the clamp on the existing IV administration set. Also, close the clamp on the short extension tubing connected to the IV catheter in the patient's arm.	
——	——	——	17. If using an electronic infusion device, remove current administration set from device. Following manufacturer's directions, insert new administration set into infusion device.	
——	——	——	18. Put on gloves. Remove the current infusion tubing from the access cap on the short extension IV tubing. Using an antimicrobial swab, cleanse access cap on extension tubing. Remove the end cap from the new administration set. Insert the end of the administration set into the access cap. Loop the administration set tubing near the site of entry, and anchor with tape (nonallergenic) close to site.	
——	——	——	19. Open the clamp on the extension tubing. Open the clamp on the administration set.	

Changing an IV Solution Container and Administration Set *(Continued)*

Excellent	Satisfactory	Needs Practice		Comments
——	——	——	20. If using an electronic infusion device, open the slide clamp, check the drip chamber of the administration set, verify the flow rate programmed in the infusion device, and turn the device to "run" or "infuse."	
——	——	——	21. If using gravity infusion, slowly open the roller clamp on the administration set and count the drops. Adjust until the correct drop rate is achieved.	
——	——	——	22. Remove equipment. Ensure patient's comfort. Remove gloves. Lower bed, if not in lowest position.	
——	——	——	23. Remove additional PPE, if used. Perform hand hygiene.	
——	——	——	24. Return to check flow rate and observe IV site for infiltration 30 minutes after starting infusion and at least hourly thereafter. Ask the patient if he or she is experiencing any pain or discomfort related to the IV infusion.	

Skill Checklists for Fundamentals of Nursing:
The Art and Science of Nursing Care, 7th edition

Name _____ Date _____

Unit _____ Position _____

Instructor/Evaluator: _____ Position _____

SKILL 40-3

Monitoring an IV Site and Infusion

Excellent	Satisfactory	Needs Practice	**Goal:** The patient remains free from complications and demonstrates signs and symptoms of fluid balance.	Comments
——	——	——	1. Verify IV solution order on MAR/CMAR with the medical order. Clarify any inconsistencies. Check the patient's chart for allergies. Check for color, leaking, and expiration date. Know the purpose of the IV administration and medications if ordered.	
——	——	——	2. *Monitor IV infusion every hour or per agency policy. More frequent checks may be necessary if medication is being infused.*	
——	——	——	3. Perform hand hygiene and put on PPE, if indicated.	
——	——	——	4. Identify the patient.	
——	——	——	5. Close curtains around bed and close door to room if possible. Explain what you are going to do to the patient.	
——	——	——	6. If an electronic infusion device is being used, check settings, alarm, and indicator lights. Check set infusion rate. Note position of fluid in IV container in relation to time tape. Teach patient about the alarm features on the electronic infusion device.	
——	——	——	7. If IV is infusing via gravity, check the drip chamber and time the drops. (Refer to Guidelines for Nursing Care 40-3 to review calculation of IV flow rates for gravity infusion.)	
——	——	——	8. Check tubing for anything that might interfere with flow. Be sure clamps are in the open position.	
——	——	——	9. Observe dressing for leakage of IV solution.	
——	——	——	10. *Inspect the site for swelling, leakage at the site, coolness, or pallor, which may indicate infiltration. Ask if patient is experiencing any pain or discomfort. If any of these symptoms are present, the IV will need to be removed and restarted at another site. Check facility policy for treating infiltration.*	
——	——	——	11. *Inspect site for redness, swelling, and heat. Palpate for induration. Ask if patient is experiencing pain. These findings may indicate phlebitis. Notify primary care provider if phlebitis is suspected. IV will need to be discontinued and restarted at another site. Check facility policy for treatment of phlebitis.*	

SKILL 40-3

Monitoring an IV Site and Infusion *(Continued)*

Excellent	Satisfactory	Needs Practice		Comments
——	——	——	12. *Check for local manifestations (redness, pus, warmth, induration, pain) that may indicate an infection is present at the site, or systemic manifestations (chills, fever, tachycardia, hypotension) that may accompany local infection at the site. If signs of infection are present, discontinue the IV and notify the primary care provider.* Be careful not to disconnect IV tubing when putting on patient's hospital gown or assisting the patient with movement.	
——	——	——	13. Be alert for additional complications of IV therapy.	
——	——	——	a. *Fluid overload can result in signs of cardiac and/or respiratory failure. Monitor intake and output and vital signs. Assess for edema and auscultate lung sounds. Ask if patient is experiencing any shortness of breath.*	
——	——	——	b. Check for bleeding at the site.	
——	——	——	14. If possible, instruct patient to call for assistance if any discomfort is noted at site, solution container is nearly empty, flow has changed in any way, or if the electronic pump alarm sounds.	

Skill Checklists for Fundamentals of Nursing:
The Art and Science of Nursing Care, 7th edition

Name _____   Date _____

Unit _____   Position _____

Instructor/Evaluator: _____   Position _____

SKILL 40-4

Changing a Peripheral Venous Access Dressing

Goal: The patient exhibits an access site that is clean, dry, and without evidence of any signs and symptoms of infection, infiltration, or phlebitis. In addition, the dressing will be clean, dry, and intact and the patient will not experience injury.

Excellent	Satisfactory	Needs Practice		Comments
——	——	——	1. Determine the need for a dressing change. Check facility policy. Gather all equipment and bring to bedside.	
——	——	——	2. Perform hand hygiene and put on PPE, if indicated.	
——	——	——	3. Identify the patient.	
——	——	——	4. Close curtains around bed and close door to room if possible. Explain what you are going to do and why you are going to do it to the patient. Ask the patient about allergies to tape and skin antiseptics.	
——	——	——	5. Put on mask and place on patient, if indicated. Put on gloves. Place towel or disposable pad under the arm with the venous access. If solution is currently infusing, temporarily stop the infusion. Hold the catheter in place with your nondominant hand and *carefully remove old dressing and/or stabilization/ securing device.* Use adhesive remover as necessary. Discard dressing.	
——	——	——	6. *Inspect IV site for presence of phlebitis (inflammation), infection, or infiltration.* Discontinue and relocate IV, if noted.	
——	——	——	7. *Cleanse site with an antiseptic solution such as chlorhexidine or according to facility policy. Press applicator against the skin and apply chlorhexidine using a back and forth friction scrub for at least 30 seconds. Do not wipe or blot. Allow to dry completely.*	
——	——	——	8. Open the skin protectant wipe. Apply the skin protectant to the site, making sure to cover at minimum the area to be covered with the dressing. Allow to dry. Place sterile transparent dressing or catheter securing/stabilization device over venipuncture site.	

SKILL 40-4

Changing a Peripheral Venous
Access Dressing *(Continued)*

Excellent	Satisfactory	Needs Practice		Comments
——	——	——	9. Label dressing with date, time of change, and initials. Loop the tubing near the site of entry, and anchor with tape (non-allergenic) close to site. Resume fluid infusion, if indicated. Check that IV flow is accurate and system is patent (Refer to Skill 40-3).	
——	——	——	10. Remove equipment. Ensure patient's comfort. Remove gloves. Lower bed, if not in lowest position.	
——	——	——	11. Remove additional PPE, if used. Perform hand hygiene.	

Skill Checklists for Fundamentals of Nursing:
The Art and Science of Nursing Care, 7th edition

Name _____   Date _____

Unit _____   Position _____

Instructor/Evaluator: _____   Position _____

Excellent	Satisfactory	Needs Practice	SKILL 40-5 **Capping for Intermittent Use and Flushing a Peripheral Venous Access Device**	
			Goal: The patient remains free of injury and any signs and symptoms of IV complications.	**Comments**
___	___	___	1. Determine the need for conversion to an intermittent access. Verify medical order. Check facility policy. Gather all equipment and bring to bedside.	
___	___	___	2. Perform hand hygiene and put on PPE, if indicated.	
___	___	___	3. Identify the patient.	
___	___	___	4. Close curtains around bed and close door to room if possible. Explain what you are going to do and why you are going to do it to the patient. Ask the patient about allergies to tape and skin antiseptics.	
___	___	___	5. Assess the IV site. Refer to Skill 40-3.	
___	___	___	6. If using an electronic infusion device, stop the device. Close the roller clamp on the administration set. If using gravity infusion, close the roller clamp on the administration set.	
___	___	___	7. Put on gloves. Close the clamp on the short extension tubing connected to the IV catheter in the patient's arm.	
___	___	___	8. Remove the administration set tubing from the extension set. Cleanse the end cap with an antimicrobial swab.	
___	___	___	9. Insert the saline flush syringe into the cap on the extension tubing. Pull back on the syringe to aspirate the catheter for positive blood return. If positive, instill the solution over 1 minute or flush the line according to facility policy. Remove syringe and reclamp the extension tubing.	
___	___	___	10. If necessary, loop the extension tubing near the site of entry, and anchor with tape (nonallergenic) close to site.	
___	___	___	11. Remove equipment. Ensure patient's comfort. Remove gloves. Lower bed, if not in lowest position.	
___	___	___	12. Remove additional PPE, if used. Perform hand hygiene.	

Skill Checklists for Fundamentals of Nursing:
The Art and Science of Nursing Care, 7th edition

Name _____ Date _____

Unit _____ Position _____

Instructor/Evaluator: _____ Position _____

Excellent	Satisfactory	Needs Practice	SKILL 40-6 **Administering a Blood Transfusion** **Goal:** The patient receives the blood transfusion without any evidence of a transfusion reaction or complication.	Comments
――	――	――	1. Verify the medical order for transfusion of blood product. Verify the completion of informed consent documentation in the medical record. Verify any medical order for pretransfusion medication. If ordered, administer medication at least 30 minutes prior to initiating transfusion.	
――	――	――	2. Gather all equipment and bring to bedside.	
――	――	――	3. Perform hand hygiene and put on PPE, if indicated.	
――	――	――	4. Identify the patient.	
――	――	――	5. Close curtains around bed and close door to room if possible. Explain what you are going to do and why you are going to do it to the patient. Ask the patient about previous experience with transfusion and any reactions. Advise patient to report any chills, itching, rash, or unusual symptoms.	
――	――	――	6. Prime blood administration set with the normal saline IV fluid. Refer to Skill 40-2.	
――	――	――	7. Put on gloves. If patient does not have a venous access in place, initiate peripheral venous access. Refer to Skill 40-1. Connect the administration set to the venous access device via the extension tubing. Refer to Skill 40-1. Infuse the normal saline per facility policy.	
――	――	――	8. Obtain blood product from blood bank according to agency policy. Scan for bar codes on blood products if required.	
――	――	――	9. Two nurses compare and validate the following information with the medical record, patient identification band, and the label of the blood product:	
――	――	――	• Medical order for transfusion of blood product	
――	――	――	• Informed consent	
――	――	――	• Patient identification number	
――	――	――	• Patient name	
――	――	――	• Blood group and type	
――	――	――	• Expiration date	
――	――	――	• Inspection of blood product for clots	

SKILL 40-6
Administering a Blood Transfusion *(Continued)*

Excellent	Satisfactory	Needs Practice		Comments
——	——	——	10. *Obtain baseline set of vital signs before beginning transfusion.*	
——	——	——	11. Put on gloves. If using an electronic infusion device, put the device on "hold." Close the roller clamp closest to the drip chamber on the saline side of the administration set. Close the roller clamp on administration set below the infusion device. Alternately, if using infusing via gravity, close the roller clamp on the administration set.	
——	——	——	12. Close the roller clamp closest to the drip chamber on the blood product side of the administration set. Remove the protective cap from the access port on the blood container. Remove the cap from the access spike on the administration set. Using a pushing and twisting motion, insert the spike into the access port on the blood container, taking care not to contaminate spike. Hang blood container on the IV pole. Open the roller clamp on the blood side of the administration set. Squeeze drip chamber until the in-line filter is saturated. Remove gloves.	
——	——	——	13. *Start administration slowly (no more than 25–50 mL for the first 15 minutes). Stay with the patient for the first 5 to 15 minutes of transfusion.* Open the roller clamp on administration set below the infusion device. Set the rate of flow and begin the transfusion. Alternately, start the flow of solution by releasing the clamp on the tubing and counting the drops. Adjust until the correct drop rate is achieved. Assess the flow of the blood and function of the infusion device. Inspect the insertion site for signs of infiltration.	
——	——	——	14. Observe patient for flushing, dyspnea, itching, hives or rash, or any unusual comments.	
——	——	——	15. After the observation period (5–15 minutes), increase the infusion rate to the calculated rate to complete the infusion within the prescribed time frame, no greater than 4 hours.	
——	——	——	16. Reassess vital signs after 15 minutes. Obtain vital signs thereafter according to facility policy and nursing assessment.	
——	——	——	17. Maintain the prescribed flow rate as ordered or as deemed appropriate based on the patient's overall condition, keeping in mind the outer limits for safe administration. Ongoing monitoring is crucial throughout the entire duration of the blood transfusion for early identification of any adverse reactions.	

Administering a Blood Transfusion *(Continued)*

Excellent	Satisfactory	Needs Practice		Comments

			18. *During transfusion, assess frequently for transfusion reaction. Stop blood transfusion if you suspect a reaction. Quickly replace the blood tubing with a new administration set primed with normal saline for IV infusion. Initiate an infusion of normal saline for IV at an open rate, usually 40 mL/hour. Obtain vital signs. Notify physician and blood bank.*	
			19. When transfusion is complete, close roller clamp on blood side of the administration set and open the roller clamp on the normal saline side of the administration set. Initiate infusion of normal saline. When all of blood has infused into patient, clamp administration set. Obtain vital signs. Put on gloves. Cap access site or resume previous IV infusion (Refer to Skills 40-1 and 40-5). Dispose of blood-transfusion equipment or return to blood bank according to facility policy.	
			20. Remove equipment. Ensure patient's comfort. Remove gloves. Lower bed, if not in lowest position.	
			21. Remove additional PPE, if used. Perform hand hygiene.	